THE HEART OF AROMATHERAPY

An Easy-to-Use Guide for Essential Oils

Andrea Butje

HAY HOUSE, INC.

Carlsbad, California • New York City
London • Sydney • Johannesburg
Vancouver • New Delhi

Published and distributed in the United States by: Hay House, Inc.: www.hayhouse.com®
Published and distributed in Australia by: Hay House Australia Pty. Ltd.: www.hayhouse.com.au
Published and distributed in the United Kingdom by: Hay House UK, Ltd.: www.hayhouse.co.uk
Published and distributed in the Republic of South Africa by: Hay House SA (Pty), Ltd.: www.hayhouse
.co.za • *Distributed in Canada by:* Raincoast Books: www.raincoast.com • *Published in India by:* Hay
House Publishers India: www.hayhouse.co.in

Indexer: Jay Kreider
Cover design: Tricia Breidenthal • *Interior design:* Bryn Starr Best

Interior photos/illustrations: illustrations used under license from Shutterstock.com except for:
Bergamot Mint: *AbbÈ H. Coste - Flore de la France (1937).*
Roman chamomile: *By Oceancetaceen - Alice Chodura - Vogtherr, M. (1898)*
Kunzea Ambigua: *M. Sorensen, Addisonia, Vol. 20*
Palmerosa: *G. E. Rumphius, Herbarium Amboinense, Vol. 5*
Palo Santo: *N. J. Jacquin, Selectarum Stirpium Americanarum Historia, vol. 2*
Piñon Pine: *C. S. Sargent, The Silva of North America, vol. 11*
Rosalina: *H. C. Andrews, The Botanist's Respository, vol. 3*
Saro: *Baillon, Adansonia, vol. 7*
Spikenard: *J. D. Hooker, Curtis's Botanical Magazine, vol. 107*

Library of Congress Cataloging-in-Publication Data

Names: Butje, Andrea, author.
Title: The heart of aromatherapy : an easy-to-use guide for essential oils / Andrea Butje.
Description: Carlsbad, California : Hay House, Inc., [2017] | Includes index.
Identifiers: LCCN 2016040445 | ISBN 9781401951610 (paperback)
Subjects: LCSH: Aromatherapy. | Essences and essential oils--Therapeutic use.
| Self-care, Health. | BISAC: HEALTH & FITNESS / Aromatherapy. | HEALTH & FITNESS / Healthy Living.
| SELF-HELP / Stress Management.
Classification: LCC RM666.A68 B88 2017 | DDC 615.3/219--dc23 LC record available at
https://lccn.loc.gov/2016040445

Tradepaper ISBN: 978-1-4019-5161-0
10 9 8 7 6 5 4 3 2 1
1st edition, January 2017

Printed in the United States of America

SUSTAINABLE
FORESTRY
INITIATIVE

Certified Sourcing
www.sfiprogram.org
SFI-01268

SFI label applies to text stock only

For my Cindy

In this vast universe, you are my home.
I love and adore you.

For the farmers and distillers

Thank you for the extraordinary commitment, love,
and hard work you put into growing the plants and
extracting our precious essential oils.
You are the foundation of the
aromatherapy profession.

Contents

Introduction

The First Time I Really Met Lavender

In the year 1995, when I was studying aromatherapy in London, I had the chance to cross the English Channel and visit a lavender distiller in Provence, France. I had never visited an essential oil distiller before, and it had always been a dream of mine. How could I say no?

My friends Rhiannon and Bob invited me to go in their tiny European car. We rolled the windows down so we could enjoy the perfect July weather, and set off toward the distillery. The smell of lavender filled the air when we were still miles away, and I took a deep breath. I had already been looking forward to this, and now I was really excited—I was actually going to meet people who distilled lavender essential oil!

I will never forget rounding the corner on that bumpy little road and seeing endless fields of lavender stretching out before me. I couldn't believe my eyes—row upon row of lush lavender plants as far as I could see! The endless expanse of purple was exquisite. It really took my breath away.

We drove along roads that wove in and out of the fields, passing roadside stalls that sold fresh and dried bundles of lavender, lavender soap, creams, body oils, mists, potpourri, and many other wonderful products, all handmade by local artisans.

The day got only more exciting when we arrived at the distillery. The stainless-steel stills had obviously been loved—they weren't new, but they were very well kept. I spent a long time talking with the two distillers, who shared their stories about growing the lavender without chemicals or pesticides, and harvesting it by hand in the early days. I stayed with them while they distilled a fresh batch of essential oil, and I couldn't believe the jaw-dropping amount of plant material they loaded into their still. I watched the distillation process, and after 1 hour and 15 minutes of distillation, the oil dripped into a clear glass container, yielding one liter of essential oil.

Just one liter!

That was the first time I really understood how concentrated a single drop of essential oil is.

The liter of oil was a thin layer on top of a much more substantial layer of liquid—the hydrosol. The hydrosol was the water they'd used in the still, which had become infused with the water-soluble components of the lavender flowers. Hydrosols that are created during essential oil distillation are pure, aromatic waters that have therapeutic properties. We washed our faces, hands, and feet with the lavender hydrosol. It was so refreshing!

The more I talked with the distillers, the more impressed I was with their work and their overall approach to life. They were in touch with the land where they had been working organically for many years. They had no website or marketing. They were simply a local, small-scale lavender farm and distillery, making and selling products to the locals, pharmacies, and people who made aromatherapy products and perfumes. I had always purchased my essential oils from companies with their own labels on the bottles, and now I realized that this small farm—and others like it around the world—was where the oils really came from.

The oil had taken on a new personality for me. It was just as gentle, relaxing, and inspiring as before, but it was no longer simply the liquid essence of the plant in a bottle. Using the oil felt like being with a friend who always left me feeling restored and uplifted. I still feel centered and calm in my heart whenever I smell lavender essential oil.

My new outlook extended into my aromatherapy studies. I took more trips to visit distillers around the world, and the more time I spent with other essential oils, the more they all began to feel like friends.

Teaching classes in the therapeutic uses of essential oils felt like a very natural development for me. In 1998, I founded Aromahead Institute, teaching classes in the art of blending and the science of essential oils.

Feeling educated about essential oils is such an empowering experience because there are so many different oils you can work with. They all offer the nourishment of the plant they are distilled from in a single drop, and education helps you understand which oils to reach for at which times. Nature works holistically . . . and so do we. When nature touches one area of your life, you can feel it in many other areas. Essential oils demonstrate this in a big way. I believe that aromatherapy is a gateway into a broader understanding of traditional healing, and a path toward healthy living.

I am still amazed when I use lavender essential oil to restore my skin after I've been exposed to the sun all day, and it helps me slip off to sleep easily. Or when I use sweet orange essential oil to ease my belly after I've eaten a little too much and feel tension I didn't even know I was carrying melt away from my muscles.

There are so many different essential oils that can help you calm down, give you more energy, ease worries and fears, help you release anxiety, soothe sore muscles, nourish skin, help you stay healthy and prevent illness, and help you recover from injuries more quickly and comfortably . . . and that's only the tip of the iceberg! Each of the oils has more than one property—just as people have more than one aspect to their personality—so when you use the oils for one purpose, you can experience multiple benefits.

Staying healthy is an ongoing process—a way of living rather than a result.

Essential oils offer a natural way to engage in this process—to care for yourself and your family, create a beautiful and comforting home, and unfold new layers of vitality and happiness. Think about how a plant can go from a seed to a flowering fruit tree that feeds many people year after year, and you'll get an idea of how essential oils can bring about transformation. The transformation can be in your heart, mind, body . . . or all three!

Essential Oils and Relaxation

Simply Profound!

Two of the most popular reasons people use essential oils are for relaxation and balance.

It seems that every day, researchers discover new reasons that stress can be harmful for your body and well-being. When you're stressed or upset, your body doesn't rest, digest, or rejuvenate as easily. Your ability to bounce back can slow down.

Tension can begin in a variety of ways. It can start physically, mentally, or emotionally, and then radiate out to affect the rest of you.

For example, if you have a difficult day at work and have to stay late, you might have a headache that evening. How did the experience of your tough day translate to head pain that night?

Your body took on your mental and emotional stress. In this case, your body might be saying, "We need to have more time off!"

The opposite is true too. Tension that starts in your body can contribute to tension in your heart and mind. If you injure a tendon in your leg, the discomfort can make you feel frustrated, overwhelmed, or afraid. On top of the pain, you can't go about your life with as much ease as you once did, so a difficult day at work will be even more of a challenge. That can add more layers to your stress.

It can become a cycle—a kind of "feedback loop" that sends stress signals from heart, to mind, to body, and back again. The longer this continues, the more out of balance you become, and the more vulnerable you are to disease and distress.

In addition to helping you feel more balanced and heal more quickly, relaxation can support you to:

1. Be more present in the moment, so you can appreciate the beauty and synchronicity in your life.

2. Listen to your body so you can sense your innate healing wisdom and take actions to guide you to vibrant health.

3. Connect with people in your life more deeply and treasure the exquisite experience of loving others.

4. Feel supported and centered during difficult circumstances. (I'm always grateful for this one.)

5. Make decisions that reflect your deepest values and dreams.

6. Have more fun!

Sometimes you can make changes in your lifestyle to reduce stress and relax more. However, it's not always possible to change your conditions. Sometimes work is just busy or you're in a transition between jobs. Sometimes you get sick or injured, and your body is healing or changing. Sometimes you're traveling too much, and jet lag gets your sleep schedule off track. These things happen, and it's not always something you can control.

This is where the essential oils come in! One of the ways the oils can support you is by helping you respond to your conditions in a more harmonious way.

Many essential oils have components that are known to offer a deep sense of relaxation. For example, one of the main components in lavender essential oil is linalool (also spelled "linalol"). A lot of research has been done showing that linalool has profound effects on the nervous system and can help people relax.

But you don't need any research to know which aromas you love, and sometimes being with an aroma you love is all it takes to help you feel relaxed and centered. After all my years of using oils, it still feels magical when I take the time to simply breathe in one of my favorite scents, and feel myself become more uplifted and calm. The aromas that affect you most deeply can be very personal to you, and it's exciting to discover your reactions to them and find the ones that give you a sense of home and comfort.

Since the oils work holistically, they can ease stress in your body, mind, and emotions.

If life is constantly go-go-go, essential oils can help you relax and move in harmony with the busy pace. (Go home from work without a headache!)

If people in your home are sick, essential oils can help your immune system stay strong so you can care for them and yourself.

If you can't sleep, you can use essential oils throughout your day to help your body and mind learn what it means to slow down and relax. When it's time for bed, they can help you unwind and get to sleep more easily.

It's easy to lose connection with yourself during stressful times—it's as though you're constantly in a state of reaction, instead of having the time to consult with your heart and sense what it wants. Like good friends, the oils help you stay connected to yourself.

Try picking a few oils that you love, and add 10 to 15 drops to an aromatherapy inhaler. An inhaler is a little lip balm–size tube with a cotton insert that absorbs essential oils. You can carry an inhaler with you in a pocket or bag, so it's very convenient. The aromas accompany you throughout the day, and any time you want to lift your mood, calm your mind, or reconnect with yourself, you can take a few deep breaths from your inhaler. Aromatherapy can be that simple, and that profound.

Different times call for different responses. What you need on a daily basis will probably be different what what you need in urgent situations. Summer and winter can affect you differently, as can morning and evening. The support you need when you're healthy is not the same as what you'll need when your body is hurting.

To know what's right for you, pay attention to how you feel and which oils make you feel your best.

about essential oils

Plants can support people in many ways. Some produce foods—fruits, vegetables, roots, leaves, herbs, and spices. Some offer shelter with their branches and materials for building homes. Some plants make wonderful medicines, or natural oils and butters that can nourish skin and hair. Some plants can also make essential oils.

The aromatic plants that produce essential oils have found a lot of different ways to store them, from wood, leaves, fruits, and roots to resins, seeds, and flowers.

Plants use their essential oils for many of the same things we can use the oils for ourselves, including fighting off infections, repelling bugs, and healing wounds.

There are several methods of obtaining essential oils from plants. Two popular ones are steam distillation and cold-pressing. All of the oils in this book are steam distilled except for the citrus oils, which are cold-pressed.

THE AROMAHEAD APPROACH TO DILUTING ESSENTIAL OILS

Essential oils are highly concentrated. When you're making aromatherapy blends with them, it's good to remember you're working with powerful substances. A little bit of essential oil really can go a long way.

It takes a huge amount of plant material to produce a small amount of essential oil. For example, it takes anywhere from 30 to 50 blossoms to produce a single drop of rose oil. Imagine four dozen roses producing one drop of essential oil.

That much plant material calls for a lot of respect, especially when it's concentrated into an essential oil.

At Aromahead Institute, we've developed a relationship to the oils that calls for using the least amount of drops necessary to accomplish your goals. We call it the Aromahead Approach. In the Aromahead Approach, essential oils are usually diluted in a carrier (a natural oil or butter) before they're applied topically to the skin. Diluting your essential oils in this way allows you to experience all the oils' benefits with less concern of negative skin or health reactions.

Here are four excellent reasons to dilute essential oils with the Aromahead Approach before applying them to your skin:

1. **Respecting the plants and the environment.** Considering how long it takes to grow the plants, and how much work goes into harvesting them and producing the oils, it makes sense to recognize essential oils as precious. Diluting the oils is one way to show respect for the entire process, and to preserve our natural resources.

2. **A little goes a long way.** Using more essential oil doesn't necessarily mean you're going to get more of its benefits. In fact, using too much of an essential oil may mean you're increasing the chances a negative reaction will occur, such as nausea or a headache.

3. **Skin irritation and allergic reactions.** Using an essential oil undiluted (or in a dilution that's too high) can potentially lead to very uncomfortable skin irritation or, on rare occasions, an allergic reaction. Read more about this and other skin reactions, including phototoxicity, in the safety guidelines.

4. **Carrier oils and butters nourish skin.** Natural carrier oils and butters, such as jojoba and cocoa butter, are nourishing and moisturizing. Since many essential oils can dry skin out if they're applied neat, carrier oils offer a lot of protection while offering their own remarkable therapeutic effects.

Does using the Aromahead Approach mean you can never use a drop of essential oil "neat" (applied directly to your skin)? No, it doesn't mean that! There are instances when a single drop of lavender, or a similar skin-friendly oil, is a good choice, such as for a bee sting.

But for everyday use, the Aromahead Approach is generally to dilute essential oils for topical use. It also calls for lower drop counts in blends for children than for adults. (You can read more about that in the safety guidelines for children on **page 15**.)

You can create different dilution ratios based on the number of drops you add to a carrier oil or butter. Our recommended dilution range for the essential oils covered in this book is 1 to 3 percent, and all of the recipes in the book stick to that range. (For specific dilution guidelines for each oil, check the safety sections in the essential oil profiles.)

There are a lot of essential oils that we don't discuss in this book, and some of those have different safety guidelines. Always be sure to check the safety information for the essential oils you're using, as some call for dilutions lower than 1 percent.

Below, you'll find a chart to make it simple to use the right number of drops to create dilution ratios from 1 to 3 percent.

There's also a chart to help you understand conversions between ounces (oz), milliliters (ml), and grams (g). In the United States, ounces are common for both liquids and solids—that is, for both volume and weight. If you're using the metric system, you'll be blending with milliliters for liquids (measuring by volume) and grams for solids (measuring by weight). Here are some helpful conversions. Some of these are rounded slightly up or down to create measurements that are easier to remember. That way you don't have to worry about measuring "half a ml," or "half a g."

Here are the Aromahead guidelines for when to blend at a 1 percent, 2 percent, or 3 percent dilution:

	1%	2%	3%
1 oz	5–6 drops	10–12 drops	15–18 drops
2 oz	10–12 drops	20–24 drops	30–36 drops
3 oz	15–18 drops	30–36 drops	45–54 drops

Ounces	Milliliters (volume)	Grams (weight)
1 oz	30 ml	28 g
2 oz	60 ml	56 g
3 oz	90 ml	84 g

- **1 percent** – Work with a 1 percent dilution for pregnant women, the elderly, and children over five years old (see the safety guidelines on **page 15** for more on using oils for kids). This percentage is also a good place to start for people who are sensitive to fragrances or chemicals.
- **2 percent** – This is a good dilution for overall skin care (although 1 percent or less is generally more appropriate for the face), and blends you're going to use on a day-to-day basis. Dilutions of 1 percent or 2 percent are nice for emotional support too.
- **3 percent** – If you're blending to support yourself through a specific short-term health concern, such as a cold or for pain relief, 3 percent is a good dilution.

When you're measuring and blending your essential oils and other ingredients, you may want to use a kitchen scale (for grams and ounces) and graduated cylinder (for milliliters). These will give you consistent measurements.

Scales come with a handy "tare" function, which allows you to set a small bowl on the scale, then "erase the bowl's weight" by setting the scale back to zero. That means that when you measure your ingredients, you're not taking the bowl's weight into account.

For recipes that call for a lot of essential oil, you can measure your essential oils by pouring them into a graduated cylinder rather than adding them to your blend drop by drop. This can save you some time and ensure a more accurate drop count, since drops can sometimes come quickly out of a bottle (and it's easy to lose count).

Another reason graduated cylinders are more accurate is because different essential oil bottles have different sizes of orifice reducers. The orifice reducer is a small insert plugged into the top of the bottle, with a tiny hole in the middle of it. It literally reduces the size of the bottle's opening so you can get small drops instead of pouring the oil out of the bottle in a stream. One orifice reducer may give you a smaller drop of oil, while another gives you a slightly bigger drop.

Another consideration is that some essential oils are thick and some are thin, so drop sizes are simply not consistent. After many years of counting essential oil drops, I've found that there are about 18 to 35 drops per ml, depending on the oil and the bottle. At Aromahead, we've settled on 25 drops per ml as a good average.

This means that if you're making a recipe that calls for 75 drops of essential oil, you can measure 3 ml of oil into your graduated cylinder instead of counting—drop by drop—to 75.

Storing Your Essential Oils

Different essential oils have different shelf lives due to a process called oxidation, which can take anywhere from months to years depending on the chemistry of the oil and the way it's stored. When an essential oil oxidizes, it has the potential to become quite skin-irritating or sensitizing.

The best way to slow down oxidation is to store your essential oils:

- In a cool, dark place
- In bottles that are closed tightly
- In bottles that are mostly full so there's little room for oxygen

Light, heat, and oxygen all speed up the process of oxidation and shorten your oils' shelf lives. Using color-tinted glass bottles and jars, like amber or cobalt blue, can help protect your oils from light and extend shelf life.

The amount that storage conditions can affect the shelf lives of your oils varies from oil to oil. A good example is orange, which has a shelf life of about one year. If you store it well, you could stretch your oil's shelf life to about two years.

The same is true for the blends you make with your oils. Store them away from light and heat, and in containers that close tightly.

It's not easy for most people to tell when an essential oil is oxidized. Your best bet is to be aware if the oil was either distilled or cold-pressed, and what its approximate shelf life is. Shelf life doesn't begin the day you purchase the oil, but the year and season the oil was produced by the distiller.

To keep track of your ingredients' shelf lives, you may want to make a list or a chart, and store it with your oils.

You might also want to purchase essential oils in smaller amounts at first, until you know which ones you love and tend to use most often. If your bottle of orange oil is still half full one year after you bought it, you might want to get a smaller bottle next time, but if you go through your lavender in less than a year, you can buy a bigger bottle.

The shelf life of any product you make depends on the shelf lives of the ingredients in it. This means that the ingredient with the shortest shelf life determines the overall shelf life of the blend. For example, let's say you make a massage oil with jojoba, lavender essential oil, and neroli essential oil. If your lavender has two years' shelf life left, but your neroli has only one year left, then your massage oil will last only one year (as long as you store it in a cool, dark place).

When you make the water-based blends in this book, such as room spritzes in water, or hydrosol blends, I recommend making them fresh every few weeks. Blends made with water-based products are more susceptible to the growth of bacteria, yeast, mold, and other things you don't want on your skin or in your environment.

When it comes to the kinds of containers you make your blends in, I prefer to use glass with essential oils. Sometimes, however, glass isn't ideal, such as when you're in the shower and your fingers are slippery. You wouldn't want to drop the bottle and have glass shatter everywhere. So for some blends, I use PET plastic, which is known to be nonreactive and resistant to leeching.

AROMATIC NOTES

It's inspiring to discover all the different aromas you can create by blending the essential oils and carriers. Sometimes the oils' individual aromas can soften when they're included in a blend. Other oils seem to stand out everywhere they go.

One perspective on creating a balanced aromatic blend is to include all three "notes"—a deep base note, a lighter top note that makes a big impression, and a middle note that brings the deep base and light top together, resulting in a "balanced" aroma.

These different notes are called:

• Top   • Middle   • Base

Essential oils' notes result from the oils' evaporation rates. Some oils have smaller and lighter molecular structures so they evaporate more quickly; others have larger molecules so they evaporate more slowly.

Top notes are bright and fresh. Eucalyptus and all of the citruses are top notes, including lime and lemon. They evaporate quickly, which is why you can smell them right away. These aromas seem to "burst out of the bottle" and greet your nose.

Middle notes are warm and radiant. They evaporate a little more slowly than top notes, so their scent will stick around a little longer. Some of the floral and spicy oils are middle notes, such as geranium and cardamom. Using them in your blends can bridge top and base notes, making the entire aroma seem "unified and layered" instead of like several different oils standing side by side.

Base notes generally have a deep, earthy, and heavy aroma. A few good examples are patchouli and vetiver. These oils lend a rich foundation to your blends. Since they don't evaporate quickly, their scent tends to linger a lot longer on your skin than the top and middle notes.

If there seems to be a lot of "aromatic space" between your top note and middle note, such as if you're using lemon and geranium, you may want to bridge those two oils with what's called a "middle-top" note. One example of a middle-top note is frankincense. Open a bottle of frankincense, and you'll be able to smell how it's eager to greet your nose (that's the top note aspect), but it also has a deeper, richer aspect (which is the middle note). There are also "middle-base" notes. A good example is ylang ylang, a middle-base that can bridge patchouli (a base note) with geranium (a middle note). This is another way you can create a balanced aroma with several essential oils.

You don't have to use top, middle, and base notes together in every blend. Blends made with only top notes are very uplifting and energizing, and blends with only base notes are deeply grounding and centering. You'll even find that most essential oils have all three notes present in and of themselves. An oil smells different when you first drop it out of the bottle than it does several hours later. This reflects the oil's top, middle, and base notes revealing themselves over time.

Learning to identify aromatic notes is so much fun! It helps you create scents that resonate with you and that can help change how you feel.

Using Essential Oils Safely

Many people will never experience a negative reaction to essential oils, but it does happen. It's not always possible to anticipate who will experience a negative reaction or what essential oils will cause it. There's no way to guarantee 100 percent safety and 0 percent risk when you're using essential oils, but you can certainly reduce your risk as much as possible. That's what the Aromahead Approach is all about.

For the 40 essential oils covered in this book, the Aromahead Approach works well. However, there are a lot of essential oils that aren't covered in this book. Some of them will work with the Aromahead Approach to safety and dilution, and others require different considerations.

For example, Robert Tisserand, one of the authors of *Essential Oil Safety*, suggests using lemongrass essential oil at less than 1 percent to avoid allergic reactions. His guideline is 0.7 percent. In a personal conversation with him, he explained to me that this lower dilution may help people avoid having an adverse or allergic reaction.

As for the essential oils covered in this book, many of them could be used in dilution percentages that don't fall within the Aromahead Approach without causing any skin reaction. Sometimes higher dilutions, or neat (undiluted) use, of an essential oil is a good choice. For example, if a child gets stung by a bee, a single drop of pure, undiluted lavender essential oil can really help to soothe the pain and swelling. (Of course, if the child is allergic to bees, another approach is necessary.)

Although there are circumstances when using essential oils neat or at a higher dilution can be a good choice, that doesn't fall within the context of this book. You'd need more education, such as essential oil chemistry, to understand when and how to use a higher dilution.

If you're interested in learning more about essential oil safety research, I highly recommend reading the book *Essential Oil Safety* by Robert Tisserand and Rodney Young. It's an excellent resource for certified aromatherapists and for those who want a more in-depth understanding of essential oil safety. You can find information on Robert and Rodney's book in the Aromatherapy Resources section, on **page 255.**

With all that in mind, let's say you want to make essential oil aromatherapy products for all your friends. (How fun!) You would want to blend specifically for each person, to be sure you're using the right dilutions and safety precautions for everyone's needs.

Here are some guidelines to follow:

Pregnancy

For your friend who is pregnant, blend with a 1 percent dilution of essential oils. The Aromahead Approach for people who are not certified aromatherapists is to stick with a few very safe oils that don't come with many precautions. Lavender (*Lavandula angustifolia*), frankincense (*Boswellia carterii*), Roman chamomile (*Chamaemelum nobile*), cedarwood (*Juniperus virginiana*), and sweet orange (*Citrus sinensis*) are a few examples. Some women choose to wait until their first trimester is over before using essential oils at all.

I recommend talking to a certified aromatherapist too, since blending for pregnant women requires more in-depth knowledge. However, these five oils are considered safe during pregnancy when used in a 1 percent dilution.

Babies and Children

There's no agreed-upon age when it's safe to start using essential oils in blends for kids' skin. The Aromahead Approach is extra cautious. Instead of essential oils, I prefer to use only hydrosols, butters, and carrier oils on children under about five years old.

Babies and young children have very sensitive skin, and essential oils can easily become overwhelming for them since every drop is very concentrated. Hydrosols, butters, and carrier oils can often give children the nudge they need toward rebalancing their health.

That's why some of the recipes in this book don't call for any essential oils at all and are still very effective. A diaper rash cream made with beeswax, argan oil, and cocoa butter can be very soothing, and a calming spray made with lavender hydrosol can work wonders when it's time for baby to go to bed. These recipes are also perfect for people who prefer not to have any essential oils in their blends, or people who have very sensitive skin. You may even find a few favorites here for yourself. The diaper rash cream is so skin-nourishing, it can actually be used as a luxurious hand cream . . . just be sure to make two separate jars and label them clearly!

The recipes that do call for essential oils are created with adults in mind. Some need to be adjusted if you want to use them for kids. That's why I offer kid-friendly versions for most of the recipes. The kid-friendly versions use less essential oil overall than the adult versions, and in cases where the oils in the adult blend don't match the Aromahead Approach for blending for children, kid-friendly oils are substituted. These include lavender, frankincense, cedarwood, sweet orange, and Roman chamomile. When correctly diluted in a carrier, these oils aren't known to cause irritation or reactions. In fact, they make excellent substitutions for almost any recipe in this book.

Once you start using essential oils for kids' skin (around age five), the Aromahead Approach is to stay with a low dilution of 1 percent. It's fun to let kids around this age help with blending, and to make blends they can use all by themselves. Kids love using inhalers and blends in spray bottles for things like helping them sleep and soothing itches from bug bites.

Store essential oils out of reach of children. If a child happens to get a hold of a bottle or blend and ingests some of the essential oil, seek immediate medical attention.

PETS

Making a safe natural product for your cat or dog requires a solid aromatherapy education. Essential oils can be toxic for cats (and personally I would never use essential oils on the fur or skin of my cats). It's also important to be careful with other small animals. This is one area where it's best to talk to a certified aromatherapist who is educated and experienced in blending essential oils for animals.

FACE CARE

When making a facial-care blend for a friend, you can use hydrosols and carrier oils and butters safely. Essential oils shouldn't go close to your eyes, and can sometimes cause irritation on the delicate skin of your face. If you do want to use essential oil in your facial care, stick with a very skin-loving oil, such as rose, frankincense, lavender, or patchouli. It's a good idea to use one single drop per 1 oz (30 ml) of your blend and see how your skin responds. I always stay at or below a 1 percent dilution for the face.

Bath Salt Blends

The bath salt blends in this book are made with salt, jojoba, and essential oils. Pay attention to your skin's responses when using essential oils in a bath. What's comfortable for you may be different from what's comfortable for other people. You may want more jojoba, less essential oil, or different essential oils from the ones in the recipes.

I suggest using about five drops of essential oil total in a bath, and when using only floral oils in the recipe, I use even less. I also recommend making your bath salts, and any blend that's going to spend time around moisture in the shower stall or tub, every few weeks.

Asthma

People with breathing difficulties can respond to essential oils in different ways, especially oils that are commonly used for respiratory support, such as eucalyptus and myrtle. Before making a blend for your friends with asthma, have them smell the oils you want to use. Make sure the oils help their chests feel open and calm, not tight and constricted.

Chemical Sensitivities

The same guidelines for asthma and breathing issues apply to people who are very sensitive to scents and chemicals, who may develop negative reactions easily. If you're going to blend for them, stick to a low dilution of 1 percent or use only carrier oils and hydrosols.

Phototoxicity

For people who spend time in the sun, stay away from blending with phototoxic essential oils. "Phototoxic" means that if you apply the essential oil to your skin and then go out in the sun (or are exposed to any UV light, such as a tanning bed), the oil will cause a burning reaction. You could develop burns, blisters, or serious discoloration. A short walk through a parking lot to your car isn't worrisome, but going for a longer walk in the sun or working in your garden is. According to Robert Tisserand and Rodney Young's book, *Essential Oil Safety*, the risk of a phototoxic reaction can linger for 18 hours after you apply the oil or blend to your skin.

The phototoxic essential oils include many of the citruses. In this book, the citruses that are *not* phototoxic include sweet orange, yuzu, and distilled lime (only *distilled* lime is not phototoxic; *cold-pressed* lime is still phototoxic).

The phototoxic oils in this book are lemon and cold-pressed lime. You can still blend with them safely for topical use on sun-exposed skin if you stick to the specific dilution ratios below:

- Lemon: 12 drops maximum per 1 oz (30 ml) of carrier oil or butter

- Cold-Pressed Lime: 4 drops maximum per 1 oz (30 ml) (Again, there's no concern if you're using distilled lime.)

Tangerine and mandarin essential oils are other citruses that are not phototoxic. They're not in any recipes in this book, but would be excellent additions to your oil collection if you'd like to have citrus oils that don't come with phototoxic concerns.

Skin Reactions

There are two main kinds of skin reactions: skin irritation and allergies. They are different reactions, but can look similar at first glance. If you have an irritation reaction to a blend, once you stop using that blend and wash the oil off the skin, the reaction usually calms right down.

If skin irritation occurs, it usually happens soon after you apply a blend or a specific essential oil. It can show up as a feeling of burning, redness, itching, or anything that makes your skin feel uncomfortable and has you saying, "Something is not right!" In this case, you can wash your skin with soap and water and then apply carrier oil to the area. Once you experience a negative reaction from an essential oil, it's a good idea to approach that oil with caution in the future. There are always substitutions for recipes that can be gentler for you.

Certain essential oils are more likely to cause skin irritation, such as the spicier oils cardamom and ginger, but any essential oil has the potential to cause it.

In an allergic reaction, your skin can remain irritated and inflamed for hours and sometimes longer. With an allergy, every time you use that same blend (or the oil causing the allergy), the reaction will flare up again.

Allergic reactions are very unpredictable, and covering them all is beyond the scope of this book. Suffice it to say if you're allergic to an essential oil, you may always be allergic to that oil and should steer clear of it.

There is certainly no guarantee that you'll have any of these reactions. Many people never do. However, it's good to approach your essential oils with respect. Using the Aromahead Approach can offer a lot of protection for your skin and reduce your chances of developing any skin reactions, especially if you'd like to use essential oils to support your skin and your health every day.

Carriers, Carrier Oils, and Butters

Using essential oils on your skin topically is a wonderful way to get their benefits! In the chapters on dilution (**page 5**) and safety (**page 13**), you read about the Aromahead Approach to diluting essential oils so you can experience their benefits while reducing your risk of negative reactions.

This chapter will introduce you to some natural carriers, carrier oils, and butters you can use for dilution.

These natural oils are also called "fatty oils" because most of them are rich with natural fatty acids that skin loves. They're also known as "fixed oils." However, most aromatherapists use the term "carrier oils," and that's what they're called in this book.

Carriers, carrier oils, and butters come from various plants. Some bases (like aloe vera gel) are present in the plant's leaves, some are pressed out of seeds (like argan oil), and others are present in the plant's fruit itself (like coconut oil). They're all known to have very nourishing effects on skin and have been used for skin care for a long time by people in the plants' native regions.

The aloe, oils, and butters in this chapter are very nourishing and offer benefits all their own. You can use them without any essential oils for skin nourishment. Try them individually so you can get to know them, or choose two or three favorites and blend them together. In the "Skin Care" chapter (**page 137**), you'll find a few wonderful recipes for making your own body butter and skin salve with some of these ingredients.

Using these nourishing oils and butters is a wonderful way to show respect to both your skin and your essential oils.

Common name: Aloe Vera Gel
Latin name: *Aloe barbadensis*
Aroma: Fresh, delicate, and not overpowering
Source: Aloe vera is a succulent and grows around the world in many countries. Its color is clear to translucent white, and it behaves more as a liquid than a gel. You'll find plenty of aloe vera products in stores, but be aware that many are processed and have added ingredients. (Here's a hint: pure aloe vera gel isn't green!)

WHY AROMATHERAPISTS APPRECIATE ALOE

Aloe vera gel is lightweight, silky, and absorbs quickly. It is effective for reducing inflammation and soothing irritation. You can also use it for helping skin heal after damage, especially after burns. Its gentle astringent nature makes it a good ingredient for natural face washes that replace soap, and if your skin tends to be dry, you can add a bit of avocado oil or follow the aloe up with a bit of moisturizing argan oil. It is a good choice for oily skin or conditions that are moist and weepy, such as blisters. Since it's not greasy or oily, it doesn't tend to get all over clothes or linens.

It's useful for:

- Nourishing very sensitive skin
- Soothing burns (cooling)
- Reducing inflammation
- Reducing irritation, including itching, redness, and rashes
- Soap-free cleansers, including shower gels and face washes

Check the shelf life when you purchase quality aloe vera gel. It's usually about one year.

argan oil

Common name: Argan Oil
Latin name: _Argania spinosa_
Aroma: Very light, toasted, nutty
Source: Argan oil comes from Morocco, where it's handmade in a traditional process. Women harvest the argan fruits and crush them between two stones. The nuts are placed in a mill along with some water, which creates a kind of "argan dough," and the dough is kneaded by hand to press out the oil. It can take 10 hours to produce a single liter of argan oil! Argan is sometimes called "liquid gold" because of its golden color and how precious it is.

WHY AROMATHERAPISTS ADMIRE ARGAN OIL

Argan oil is light, silky, and smooth. It's been shown to have high levels of vitamin E, antioxidants, and essential fatty acids, which explains its talent for soothing irritation and nourishing skin. Argan oil does not feel oily or greasy, does not clog pores, and is a good choice for a facial moisturizer. It's often used to nourish dry nails and hair, and is popular for mature skin. You can even use it as a face wash instead of soap.

Argan oil is nourishing to areas of your skin that need a luxurious, loving kind of attention. Melted with body butters and beeswax, it helps to create a soft and luxurious blend for the skin.

Use it in blends for:

- Healing, nourishing, and protecting skin from day to day
- Softening hair, brittle nails, and dry skin
- Supporting skin as it ages
- Nourishing very sensitive skin
- Reducing inflammation
- Reducing irritation, including itching and redness
- Soap-free cleansers, including face washes

Argan oil's shelf life is about two years.

Common name: Avocado Oil

Latin name: *Persea gratissima*

Aroma: Delicate, fresh, and similar to the ripe fruit with an earthy, slightly nutty scent

Source: Avocado trees like sunny, tropical, and Mediterranean climates. The oil is cold-pressed from the fruit. Organic, unrefined avocado oil is rich in chlorophyll, so it has a distinctive dark green color. When the oil is refined, the chlorophyll is removed and the oil looks pale yellow. The raw kind has more to offer your skin.

avocado oil

WHY AROMATHERAPISTS LOVE AVOCADO OIL

Avocado oil is rich with essential fatty acids and is deeply moisturizing. It can help skin retain its natural moisture, and is good at penetrating the first few layers of skin to make it feel supple and nourished through and through. Avocado oil is often used in blends to improve skin's elasticity, and to reduce the appearance of scars and stretch marks. If soap tends to dry or irritate your skin, you can use avocado oil as a cleanser instead.

Avocado oil lends a rich green color to your blends, so be sure they won't stain light-colored clothing or linens.

When avocado oil is cold, it may become cloudy and congealed with deposits visible in the liquid. It may solidify. It will return to its clear liquid form when it's been at room temperature for a while. Avocado oil turns from green to brown as it gets older.

Use it in blends for:

- Healing, nourishing, and protecting skin from day to day
- Softening hair, brittle nails, and dry skin
- Supporting skin as it ages
- Nourishing very sensitive skin
- Caring for existing skin issues, such as scars and stretch marks
- Reducing inflammation
- Reducing irritation, including itching and redness
- Soap-free cleansers, including face washes

Avocado oil's shelf life is about one year.

Beeswax

Common name: Beeswax
Latin name: _Cera alba_
Aroma: Rich, honey-like
Source: Bees _(Apis mellifera)_ produce beeswax naturally when making their honeycombs. Once the honey is harvested, the honeycomb can be boiled in hot water. As the floating wax cools and solidifies, it's easily separated from the water.

WHY AROMATHERAPISTS BUZZ ABOUT BEESWAX

Beeswax is used for adding firmness to aromtherapy butters. Melting beeswax with liquids such as avocado oil or jojoba wax will produce a soft balm or firm salve, depending on how much beeswax you add. It helps you create rich, thick body butters that feel silky on skin. It's also used to help skin retain moisture (which makes it a humectant) and can soften very dry, chapped areas.

It is rich in vitamin A (which is important if skin cells are to develop healthily), acts as an antioxidant, and soothes irritation, including inflammation.

Use it in blends for:

- Healing, nourishing, and protecting skin from day to day
- Softening brittle nails and dry skin
- Reducing inflammation
- Reducing irritation, including itching and redness
- Caring for existing skin issues, such as scars and stretch marks

Beeswax has an exceptionally long shelf life, and can last more than 20 years when stored in a closed container in a cool environment.

Common name: Cocoa Butter
Latin name: *Theobroma cacao*
Aroma: Chocolatey, rich, warm
Source: Cacao trees can grow in any tropical climate. The firm, solid butter is obtained by pressing cacao seeds that have been fermented, washed, dried, and then roasted. Quality cocoa butter is organic and unrefined, and has a pale yellow tint to it.

WHY AROMATHERAPISTS CHERISH COCOA BUTTER

Cocoa butter is rich with skin-loving fatty acids and vitamin E, and it acts as an antioxidant. Its texture is very firm, smooth, and a bit powdery on the surface when it's solid, and it melts into a silky liquid on your skin. It is often used to restore very dry, cracked skin and to replenish aging skin. It is deeply moisturizing, nourishing, and protective.

Cocoa butter can help you make rich, luxurious body butters. It won't add as much firmness as beeswax, but it can serve to enhance the "firm factor" of your blends. Plus, it adds the aroma of chocolate!

Use cocoa butter for:

- Healing, nourishing, and protecting skin from day to day
- Brittle nails and dry skin
- Supporting skin as it ages
- Nourishing very sensitive skin
- Caring for existing skin issues, such as scars and stretch marks
- Reducing inflammation
- Reducing irritation, including itching and redness

Cocoa butter has a shelf life of about one year. If stored in a cold place, it can last longer.

Carriers, Carrier Oils, and Butters

Coconut oil

Common name: Coconut Oil
Latin name: *Cocos nucifera*
Aroma: Tropical, delicious coconut
Source: Palm trees love hot, humid, tropical climates. Coconut oil is cold-pressed from the flesh of the coconut. It is most effective when it's raw, unrefined, unfractionated, organic, and "virgin." There is a lot of coconut oil commercially available, so it's helpful to know what to look for when you're buying it. (Here's a hint: fractionated coconut oil usually doesn't have that familiar coconut scent.)

WHY AROMATHERAPISTS TREASURE COCONUT OIL

Coconut oil is used to calm irritation, including itching and redness, and skin loves its high content of saturated fatty acids. It does not clog pores and is generally safe for very sensitive skin. Use it for moisturizing and protecting skin, especially for skin conditions that need special attention. Coconut oil is rich but not heavy. You can cook with it or eat it raw by the spoonful. In aromatherapy blends, coconut oil is wonderfully moisturizing, nourishing, and protective for skin.

In cold temperatures, coconut oil is more of a solid. In warmer temperatures (above 76° F [24°C]), it's a liquid.

Use it in blends for:

- Healing, nourishing, and protecting skin from day to day
- Softening hair, brittle nails, and dry skin
- Supporting skin as it ages
- Nourishing very sensitive skin
- Reducing inflammation
- Reducing irritation, including itching and redness

Coconut oil has a shelf life of about two years.

Common name: Jojoba, Jojoba Wax
Latin name: *Simmondsia chinensis*
Aroma: Faint, sweet, barely detectable
Source: Jojoba is an evergreen shrub that grows in dry areas. Its seeds look a little like coffee beans, and when they're cold-pressed, they yield up to 60 percent of themselves as liquid wax.

WHY AROMATHERAPISTS ADORE JOJOBA

Jojoba is often called an oil, but it's actually a liquid wax. Its chemical structure is similar to the natural oily substance skin produces to protect itself (which is called "sebum"). It's nourishing and gentle for very sensitive skin. Jojoba moisturizes skin and hair, and protects skin against irritation, chapping, and itching.

Jojoba solidifies in cold temperatures, but it returns to liquid form easily.

Jojoba's aroma is quite subtle and can easily be infused with other scents. Vanilla-infused jojoba, neroli-infused jojoba, and coffee flower–infused jojoba are a few popular varieties you'll find. Infused jojoba makes a beautiful base for natural perfumes, either alone or with essential oils added.

Use it in blends for:

- Healing, nourishing, and protecting skin from day to day
- Softening hair, brittle nails, and dry skin
- Supporting skin as it ages
- Nourishing very sensitive skin
- Caring for existing skin issues, such as scars and stretch marks
- Reducing inflammation
- Reducing irritation, including itching and redness
- Balancing skin

To add to its magic, jojoba does not go rancid (a benefit of being a wax, not an oil), and can extend the shelf lives of your blends. If you blend an essential oil with a three-year shelf life into jojoba, that blend will last three years—the essential oil itself determines the shelf life of the entire blend.

Trauma Oil

Trauma oil is a blend of three herbs infused in a carrier oil. The herbs are arnica, St. John's wort, and calendula, and the carrier is usually olive oil. The herbs are known for their abilities to relieve pain and inflammation, which makes trauma oil an ideal ingredient for blends intended to soothe injuries and support recovery. Trauma oil is also skin-nourishing, which makes it safe for long-term use.

The shelf life depends on the carrier oils used as a base but is usually around a year.

Castile Soap

Castile soap is made of all-natural vegetable oils. It's traditionally made with olive oil, but there are many modern recipes for castile soap that include other oils and butters, such as shea butter and avocado oil. You can find it in bar form, but most recipes (including the ones in this book) that call for castile soap are talking about the liquid version.

Pure, quality castile soap doesn't include any synthetic substances, and is known for being very gentle for sensitive skin. It's a good ingredient in homemade hand soaps, shower gels, natural cleaning blends, and other cleansing aromatherapy products. Castile soap doesn't typically have a scent of its own, so it makes for an unobtrusive cleansing base for essential oils.

The word "castile" is used because the soap is said to have first been made in the Castile region of Spain. The shelf life depends on the ingredients in the soap, but is generally about two years.

Salts

Bath salts with essential oils can help to relieve tension. Salt scrubs are used for softening skin and circulation, and they offer gentle exfoliation at the same time. You can also use salts in some natural cleaning blends to add an abrasive element.

There are a lot of varieties of salt you can use. Epsom salt is especially good for long warm baths that relieve sore muscles. Dead Sea salt is rich with nutrients and minerals that skin loves.

I like to use pink Himalayan salt, which is mined in the Himalayas and has a lovely warm pink hue to it. Like Dead Sea salt, pink Himalayan salt is rich with minerals that can help skin feel very nourished. Most of the recipes with salt in this book call for pink Himalayan salt, but you can use any salt you prefer.

Lotion and Cream

Some recipes in this book involve blending essential oils into natural, unscented lotion or cream, which absorbs more quickly than carrier oils and butters. These recipes don't require you to actually make your own lotion or cream. Instead, you can purchase unscented lotion or cream ready-made from companies that sell natural, organic butters and oils, and who blend their own lotions and creams with the ingredients they sell. Using these products makes it simple for you to blend your essential oils into a ready-made, skin-soothing base.

Lotions and creams are made with oils, butters, and water-based ingredients. Lotion is lighter because it has more water-based ingredients in it than cream.

Check with your supplier for the shelf life of your lotion or cream.

Essential Oil Profiles

Common name: Basil, Sweet Basil, Basil ct. linalool
Latin name: *Ocimum basilicum* ct. linalool
Aroma: Herbal and sweet, reminiscent of licorice
Aromatic note: Top

BASIL'S TALENTS

Basil ct. linalool is good for helping you relax and focus at the same time. It's a reliable choice if you feel stressed, tense, or anxious—even if you're extremely busy. At the end of your day, basil can give you the calm, quiet confidence that you've done your best.

It's also very skin-nourishing, so you can use it in topical blends for concentration and meditation. A body oil with basil ct. linalool can help you release mental chatter and focus on the pleasure of the moment.

You can reach for your bottle of basil if you feel distracted by tightness lingering in your shoulders, neck, or belly. It's also a wonderful essential oil for digestion blends, where it combines well with lime, cardamom, and Roman chamomile to ease stomach discomfort. Basil ct. linalool's skin-nourishing presence can be especially helpful when paired with the spicier, potentially irritating cardamom.

Basil also offers a lot of help for respiratory issues. Constantly coughing or sniffling can break your concentration and interrupt your "flow," and basil can help to soothe coughs and break up mucus so you can focus on your day. It blends well with eucalyptus, although it has a softer touch.

Use basil ct. linalool in blends for:

- Focus and relaxation
- Respiratory support
- Calming skin inflammation
- Soothing sore muscles

- Easing painful joints
- Clearing mucus and congestion
- Relieving headaches
- Supporting digestion

BASIL'S "PEACE OF MIND" ZEN SHOP

Basil ct. linalool has always been impressed with the way connecting with ourselves can help us be more present and get more done. It's what you can experience when you cut out distractions and become absorbed in a task. Time seems to flow more freely, and you seem to be more productive than ever.

When Basil realized it had a talent for helping people be more present, it opened a chain of stores to expand its influence. Basil sells tools to help stimulate people's minds, enhance focus and productivity, and remove distractions. Some of its products are technological, such as apps that remind you to pause and take a few deep breaths throughout the day. Others are natural therapeutic products that can make you feel healthier and more connected with the moment.

One thing that attracts people to Basil's store is the beautiful aroma drifting out of the doors. That's because Basil loves to run a diffuser with a blend to help people breathe deeply. It also has a "head massage" area where people like to sit and relax while Basil massages their heads, necks, and aching joints in their hands and feet.

Basil knows that many people on tight schedules come to its shop on their lunch breaks. They eat quickly, then rush over to Basil for a little "lunchtime zen." Basil offers them a digestion cream to use while it helps them feel centered.

When people go into Basil ct. linalool's store, they immediately feel taken care of and at peace.

BASIL'S SAFETY TIPS

Basil is a good example of an essential oil that has multiple chemotypes, which have different therapeutic uses and safety considerations. (Read more about chemotypes on **page 109**.) A few other chemotypes are basil ct. estragole and basil ct. eugenol. The chemotype used in this book is basil ct. linalool (a more gentle chemotype for the skin). Based on the chemistry, Robert Tisserand and Rodney Young, authors of *Essential Oil Safety*, suggest staying under a 3% dilution when blending with basil ct. linalool.

Common name: Bergamot Mint
Latin name: *Mentha citrata*
Aroma: Warm, fresh, and fruity, with light hints of mint at the edges of the aroma
Aromatic note: Middle-Top

BERGAMOT MINT'S EXPERTISE

Bergamot mint has been shown to have a very calming effect on the nervous system.

Its aroma also has an uplifting aspect, so it can help you feel energized and centered at the same time. Try a few drops in a diffuser to relax, feel inspired, and breathe deeply.

Deep breaths of bergamot mint can help you feel healthier. It calms inflammation, including the kind that can flare up in the respiratory system, and supports your body during an infection. You can use it in diffusers and inhalers, and in blends for topical application, where it combines peppermint's cooling effects with the radiant, uplifting effects of sweet orange.

Like peppermint and sweet orange, bergamot mint also works well in blends for digestion and nausea. Blend it into a belly oil or inhaler, and reach for your blend as often as you need to help your belly feel calm and your muscles relax. You'll find it helpful for a variety of things that can upset your stomach—from eating something that doesn't agree with you, to getting a touch of motion sickness, to experiencing "nervous butterflies" in your belly due to stress.

You can use bergamot mint for:

- Respiratory support
- Clearing mucus and congestion
- Soothing sore muscles
- Supporting digestion
- Easing nausea
- Feeling motivated and inspired

BERGAMOT MINT'S "UPLIFT" YOGA STUDIO

Bergamot Mint always knew it wanted to run its own yoga studio.

It has such a peaceful, inspiring nature, and it loves staying healthy. Yoga is the perfect way for Bergamot Mint to combine its loves for health, breathing, relaxation, and emotional well-being. It calls its yoga studio "Uplift."

The "Uplift" yoga studio is known for the way its classes never fail to make people feel peaceful and happy. Students always walk out with smiles on their faces, and say they feel like they're glowing. (Its most popular class is called "Go with the Glow!") Bergamot Mint offers classes throughout the day, but its evening classes are so popular that it had to expand its schedule.

Sometimes it offers a light, community-oriented dinner after its last evening class. It serves food that's very easy to digest because it knows everyone is going to go home and fall into bed right away. Everyone sleeps peacefully after an evening class with Bergamot Mint.

Bergamot Mint loves using essential oils all around its yoga studio. It diffuses different blends during classes to help people feel calm and flow through their poses with ease. During cold and flu season, it diffuses blends that cleanse the air and help everyone breathe a little more clearly, and it passes around free inhalers to help people stop sniffling and sneezing. It also makes a body oil for one of its specialty classes (called "Muscle Massage Yoga") to soothe students' muscles when they're having trouble with certain poses. It even makes its own essential oil foam hand soap.

Bergamot Mint's yoga students have come to think of its studio as a second home, and always feel happy and welcome there.

BERGAMOT MINT'S SAFETY TIPS

Bergamot mint has a similar chemistry to lavender and is very skin-friendly.

BEHIND THE BOTTLE
ESSENTIAL OIL DISTILLERS

My passion for working with and supporting essential oil distillers began in 1998. Since then, I've been visiting essential oil distillers around the world, learning about their work, and connecting them with companies who want to buy essential oils directly from distillers.

All of the distillers I've worked with are small-scale, independently owned businesses, and many are farmers who live on the very land where they cultivate their plants. Others practice wild-crafting (also known as wild harvesting). They all take pride in using the most natural methods they can, not exposing their plants to chemical treatments, and producing pure, high-quality essential oils. Their work truly is a labor of love, as most of the consumers who use their oils have no idea who actually grows the plants and produces the oils. Most people don't see the amount of work that goes into farming and harvesting, and the attention to detail that goes into the art of distilling and cold-pressing essential oils.

Getting to know these artisans adds many layers of meaning to my experience of essential oils, and to the way I teach about them at Aromahead Institute.

When I hold a bottle of lavender from Greece in my hand, I feel connected to the island of Crete, where my friends Gill and Derek have created a remarkable farm growing lavender and olive trees. When I hold a bottle of patchouli, I'm reminded of the exotic beauty of the Seychelles islands, where patchouli once grew in abundance but is now a rare treat to find. That little bottle brings to mind the big smile of my friend Mustafa, who is working to reestablish patchouli distillation on the islands.

Knowing the people who grew the plants and produced the bottle of oil in my hand truly deepens my sense of the aromatherapy community and my commitment to the plants that give us these precious oils.

Common name: Black Spruce
Latin name: *Picea mariana*
Aroma: Coniferous, fresh, and warm
Aromatic note: Top-Middle

BLACK SPRUCE'S SKILLS

Black spruce essential oil can stir up "stuck energy." This means it's a good oil to reach for when you're feeling sluggish, and want to feel more healthy and vibrant. I especially like using black spruce essential oil during the cold, dark months of the year. Sometimes people's energy can feel less vibrant at these times, and black spruce is a very encouraging oil.

Black spruce has a helpful presence in blends for soothing respiratory issues and "sprucing up" your energy. It can support you through colds, the flu, coughs, and allergies. It's good at reducing inflammation and clearing away mucus, so it's right at home in blends meant to be breathed in, such as diffuser blends or aromatherapy inhalers. If you suffer from allergies, using black spruce in a diffuser can offer ongoing support, while helping to keep your energy up throughout the day.

Sore muscles and joints respond well to black spruce. It can ease swelling and help to calm muscle spasms. In topical blends, such as body oils and butters, it has a rejuvenating, restorative effect. Black spruce is an excellent choice for soothing aches and pains that come along with being sick.

Black spruce is ideal for:

- Respiratory support
- Clearing mucus and congestion
- Calming inflammation
- Soothing sore muscles
- Calming muscle spasms, including coughs
- Staying healthy and vibrant in winter, and anytime people around you are sick

BLACK SPRUCE'S WILD FOREST APOTHECARY

On the edge of a small Canadian village, there's a trail that leads up into an evergreen forest. The path takes you through the woods and over bridges that cross streams. After a refreshing walk, you'll find yourself at a little cabin with a sign that says "Black Spruce's Wild Forest Apothecary."

The locals come to Black Spruce for its natural therapeutic butters and oils to soothe all kinds of complaints, especially respiratory issues and body aches. Its most popular products are ready-made on its shelves, but Black Spruce especially likes to make custom blends for people. If you have a cold and cough that feels like it's coming from your chest, Black Spruce will make you a different blend than for a cold that feels like it's living in your head. Black Spruce will sit you down by its warm wood stove, pour you a cup of tea, and make your personal blend while you wait.

At Black Spruce's Wild Forest Apothecary, there are always bundles of dried herbs hanging up, a pot of tea brewing, and bowls of natural resins for sale. It's always burning a woodsy incense or diffusing an essential oil blend that helps you breathe easily.

The Apothecary doors are always open because it wants to be there around the clock if you need anything. Feel free to stop by and feel better!

BLACK SPRUCE'S SAFETY TIPS

Before using black spruce essential oil for someone who suffers from asthma or another respiratory disorder, have them smell the lid of the oil's bottle. If it makes their chest feel a little tight or constricted, use another oil for them. (Cedarwood is a good choice.) If it makes their chest feel more open, go ahead and see how a low dilution of black spruce makes them feel.

Common name: Cardamom
Latin name: *Elettaria cardamomum*
Aroma: Warm and spicy, with a fresh note that might remind you of eucalyptus, but sweeter
Aromatic note: Middle

CARDAMOM'S FLAIR

Cardamom essential oil offers excellent support for digestion. A few drops in a cream or body oil can give you such a feeling of comfort if you overindulge in dinner or a decadent dessert. It's known to calm nausea, belly cramps, and gas. Rub the blend into your belly and lower back.

Cardamom is also helpful for reducing inflammation and pain. Soothing inflammation is always a step in the right direction toward pain relief. It has a supportive, warming presence in blends for sore joints, tense muscles, and other body aches.

In blends for topical application, it's a good idea to balance cardamom's spicy presence with some very skin-loving oils, such as lavender or Roman chamomile (which can also help with digestion).

Cardamom essential oil smells delicious, comforting, and uplifting—a nice perk when it's used in diffuser blends or inhalers. Its presence helps to encourage circulation and break up congestion, which makes it effective for calming respiratory issues. You'll need only a few drops. Cardamom is a spicy essential oil, and too much can be a bit sharp for mucous membranes.

You can use cardamom for:

- Respiratory support
- Clearing mucus and congestion
- Reducing swelling
- Soothing sore muscles and joints
- Encouraging circulation and warmth
- Supporting digestion
- Easing nausea
- Feeling comforted, energized, and uplifted

CARDAMOM'S SWEETNESS 'N' SPICE CAFÉ

Cardamom wants you to enjoy all the sweetness life has to offer. That's why it opened a dessert café!

Step into Cardamom's Sweetness 'n' Spice Café, and you'll immediately notice the delicious aroma of all the good things cooking. Cardamom diffuses a supportive blend of essential oils to help its guests breathe easily and feel comfortable. Its café is a little corner of the neighborhood where you can settle in, release stress and tension, and relax.

Cardamom loves indulging in life, but it also knows how easy it is to *over*indulge. It makes aromatic belly creams that can really help if you eat a little too much. People also use its creams for nausea, nervous tension, and gas.

Cardamom always seems to know when you need a little sweetness, and when you need to pull back a bit. It's found the perfect balance between making desserts with the spice and using the essential oil for soothing creams and diffuser blends.

Take a seat in the dessert café and stay to chat with Cardamom as long as you like. A good talk with Cardamom can make you feel at home and put everything in perspective. As Cardamom would say, "Life is short, eat dessert first!"

CARDAMOM'S SAFETY TIPS

Cardamom can sometimes cause skin irritation, so you can stick with a low dilution (1 percent is good) if you're using it in blends for topical application. It's also helpful to balance cardamom with other skin-supportive essential oils and carriers.

Cardamom is a strong oil (in a similar way to eucalyptus) and is not my preference for young children, especially not in blends applied near their faces.

Common name: Cedarwood
Latin name: *Juniperus virginiana*
Aroma: Fresh, woodsy, and sweet
Aromatic note: Base

CEDARWOOD'S STRENGTHS

Cedarwood essential oil has a strongly steady, reassuring presence. It can offer strength when you're feeling sick, or if you can't seem to relax. Its soft, woody aroma can both open your breathing and comfort you, and it's so gentle that it's one of my favorite essential oils to use with kids.

Cedarwood is an amazing substitute for many strong respiratory oils, such as eucalyptus and tea tree. If you don't have one of those oils on hand or feel they're too strong, you can use cedarwood instead. This allows you to make a lot of respiratory blends safely for children. Diffusing cedarwood before bedtime or as a child falls asleep can help them breathe more easily and feel secure.

Cedarwood is also great for sore muscles and is very skin-loving. It can help small cuts and scrapes heal. Topical blends with cedarwood can support you during an infection and help you relax as you get well.

Cedarwood's overall presence is sheltering. Emotionally, it offers a peaceful sense of confidence.

Turn to it for:

- Daily skin care
- Rejuvenating damaged skin
- Soothing skin irritation
- Respiratory support
- Clearing mucus and congestion
- Tightness in your chest
- Helping to clear infections
- Calming inflammation
- Feeling relaxed and uplifted
- Soothing the nervous system
- Repelling insects
- Blends for children
- Refreshing closets and drawers

CEDARWOOD'S ELEMENTARY EDUCATION PROJECT

Cedarwood loves taking care of people, especially children, and making sure they feel safe and healthy. It has a real gift for supporting kids in an all-natural, organic way and wants to be sure everyone else has the knowledge to do the same.

So it started a business talking to nurses, teachers, and caretakers at elementary schools, helping them use more natural "first-aid" techniques.

Most nurses and teachers like to keep a small stock of Cedarwood's blends for common issues, such as bug bites, bruises, and anxiety. They also like that they can make blends on the spot for each child's needs.

Now when a child falls down on the playground, the school nurse can make one of Cedarwood's blends to reduce the possibility of infection and soothe pain, and the child can take the salve home.

Nurses can also make inhalers for kids with allergies. Kids love these because inhalers are easy and fun to use, and adults love that there's no mess and nobody else smells the essential oils.

Cedarwood loves the moments when knowledge "clicks" for people, and they realize that once they understand how to blend safely, they can get creative and make unique blends for each child and each situation. A blend to reduce allergies can also inspire peace and calm, and a blend to soothe a bee sting can offer emotional comfort.

Cedarwood's recipes for kids use very safe ingredients that don't cause reactions or irritation, but the biggest reason kids like them is because they smell so good!

CEDARWOOD'S SAFETY TIPS

Cedarwood (*Juniperus virginiana*) is considered a very safe oil. Some sources recommend avoiding it during pregnancy, but they have probably confused *Juniperus virginiana* with *Juniperus sabina*, which does come with those precautions.

What's in a (Latin) Name?

Plants that produce essential oils grow all over the world. Some grow in the wild, and some are cultivated by small-scale farmers and distillers. Since they're so international, the plants and their oils might have different names they're commonly known by from country to county. Helichrysum, for example, is also called "everlasting," and "immortelle." If you picked up a bottle of "immortelle" essential oil, you might not realize it's the same oil as helichrysum until you saw the genus and species of the plant it was obtained from—its Latin name. The Latin name is always *italicized*. The genus is capitalized and the species is in lowercase, as in *Lavandula angustifolia* (lavender).

Another good example of why it's important to check the Latin names of your essential oils are the chamomiles. There are many species of chamomile, including German chamomile (*Matricaria recutita*), Roman chamomile (*Chamaemelum nobile*), and cape chamomile (*Eriocephalus punctulatus*). Although the plants are all commonly called "chamomile," they produce very different essential oils.

chamomile (German)

Common name: German Chamomile
Latin name: _Matricaria recutita_
Aroma: Herbal, slightly fruity, and woody
Aromatic note: Middle-Base

GERMAN CHAMOMILE'S GENIUS

German chamomile's impressive ability to calm inflammation has been well researched. It has a tender yet persistent effect, continuously calming pain and introducing comfort instead. It feels cool on sunburns, especially when combined with lavender and helichrysum in aloe vera gel.

Since it's also nourishing for skin, German chamomile is a good choice for long-term pain relief and body oils meant for daily use, as well as for easing acute pain like bruises and bee stings.

You'll get the best of German chamomile's effects if you apply it in a topical blend right where it's needed, rather than using it around you in products like diffuser blends or linen sprays. It's also a precious and pricey essential oil—another reason to save it for topical blends. Just be aware that the oil has a deep blue-green color that may stain light-colored clothing or linens.

German chamomile essential oil is excellent in blends for kids over five years old. If you're blending for younger children, German chamomile hydrosol is a gentler option. You can blend German chamomile and lavender hydrosols together to create a wonderfully soothing skin spray for issues like diaper rash, bug bites, stings, burns, and small scrapes.

Use German chamomile essential oil for:

- Daily skin care
- Rejuvenating damaged skin
- Soothing skin irritation
- Reducing swelling
- Soothing sore muscles and joints
- Relieving pain, including sunburns
- Bug bites and stings

Use German chamomile hydrosol for:

- Skin-care blends for small children and babies

GERMAN CHAMOMILE'S NATURAL PARENTS BLOG

German Chamomile wanted to raise its children in a very natural lifestyle—with minimal exposure to chemicals, relying on healthy foods and healing techniques.

As German Chamomile learned more about natural parenting, it started keeping track of things on an online blog . . . which quickly gained a big following! Before long, German Chamomile began including recipes and advice not only for parenting, but for natural living and self-care as well.

Parents love German Chamomile's natural approach to pain relief. It has a real talent for soothing bumps, bruises, cuts, scrapes, and anxious emotions that come along with these accidents. In response to popular demand, it created a blend that helps soothe sunburns for kids who spend a little too long playing outside.

German Chamomile knows that kids can go through periods where they have trouble sleeping . . . and that means parents can have trouble sleeping too. So it has a whole section of its website dedicated to healthy, natural rest and relaxation. You'll find recipes for body oils and sleep spritzes to use around a baby's crib and blankets. It even sells several blends of chamomile tea.

GERMAN CHAMOMILE'S SAFETY TIPS

German chamomile is generally considered a gentle oil, but according to Robert Tisserand and Rodney Young, authors of *Essential Oil Safety*, it could potentiate the actions of some antidepressants. German chamomile could also have a drug interaction with codeine and tamoxifen.

chamomile (Roman)

Common name: Roman Chamomile
Latin name: *Chamaemelum nobile, Anthemis nobilis*
Aroma: Warm and sweet, with herbal and fruity notes, similar to apples in the sun
Aromatic note: Middle-Top

ROMAN CHAMOMILE'S RADIANCE

Roman chamomile essential oil is calming and reassuring. It can have this effect on your emotions and your body, and it really shines when it's used for both simultaneously.

In addition to having a deeply soothing effect on the nervous system, Roman chamomile has traditionally been used to relieve pain. Its abilities to calm inflammation and spasms are hints as to how it can be supportive in this way. It's excellent for soothing stress and tension, skin irritation, sore muscles and joints, and especially abdominal pain.

Roman chamomile is ideal for digestion and nausea. It's strong enough to ease muscle cramps, and gentle enough that you can use it in topical belly creams and oils as often as you need to. It's so gentle that I even trust it with children who are complaining that their bellies hurt. The aroma is not overwhelming, the oil does not irritate sensitive skin, and 5 to 6 drops in 1 oz (30 ml) of carrier oil can be very effective.

It's also an ideal choice for blends that help calm anxiety and send you off to sleep peacefully. Diffuser blends and inhalers are good ways to use it. Try it with sweet orange, patchouli, and ylang ylang.

Use Roman chamomile in blends for:

- Soothing skin irritation
- Calming inflammation
- Soothing sore muscles
- Calming muscle spasms and cramps
- Supporting digestion
- Easing nausea
- Feeling relaxed and uplifted

ROMAN CHAMOMILE'S RELAXING RIVER BOAT TOURS

If you'd like a little time-out to rest, relax, and take in some scenery, Roman Chamomile has just the thing for you: a relaxing river boat tour.

Roman Chamomile loves peace and quiet. It will take you and a few other guests on a small boat with a canopy, gliding peacefully down a smooth river shaded by tall trees. The water is always calm—no waves to make anyone nauseous or seasick. Your stress, worries, and any muscle tension will melt away, including that persistent tension headache.

Children are especially welcome on Roman Chamomile's river cruise. They love watching otters and fish in the water, and the soothing motion of the boat makes kids feel calm and safe. They might even fall asleep in their seats!

In the middle of every river cruise, Roman Chamomile serves a light, easy-to-digest dinner and cups of warm, aromatic herbal tea. (You get as many refills as you like!) On the small chance that someone does develop a bit of an upset stomach, Roman Chamomile has handmade belly butters and creams for digestion and nausea.

After your dinner, you'll get a surprise . . . Roman Chamomile has a massage therapist friend who moves quietly from guest to guest, giving everyone a relaxing shoulder and neck massage. (A lot of people say this is their favorite part.)

You'll have no trouble sleeping that night, remembering the soothing music and the calm waters, but you might have trouble not returning tomorrow for another cruise!

ROMAN CHAMOMILE'S SAFETY TIPS

The only safety tip is to be sure you're using the right kind of chamomile. There are many different species, and it's easy to pick up the wrong one. Look for the Latin name *Chamaemelum nobile* or *Anthemis nobilis*.

eucalyptus

Common name: Eucalyptus
Latin name: *Eucalyptus radiata, Eucalyptus globulus*
Aroma: Medicinal, fresh, and penetrating (which means it's bright, sharp, and infuses your senses)
Aromatic note: Top

EUCALYPTUS'S GENIUS

There may be no other essential oil more well-known for supporting healthy breathing than eucalyptus. It's famous for its ability to clear congestion, reduce mucus, and support every aspect of your respiratory system.

A good deal of research has been done on eucalyptus essential oil, and it's been found to have properties that increase circulation, reduce inflammation, ease pain, and help the body clear out mucus. True to its reputation for respiratory support, eucalyptus shines when it's inhaled. That's when it can get right to the "scene of the action"! Turn to it when you want to decongest and loosen up sensations of tightness in your chest or head.

Eucalyptus is comforting in topical blends to help soothe muscles while you're recovering from an infection. It reduces inflammation in muscles as well as it does in the respiratory system, and its cooling effect is on par with that of peppermint.

In general, it's as though eucalyptus is telling your body to open up, take a deep breath, and let go. You can turn to eucalyptus for:

- Respiratory support
- Clearing mucus and congestion
- Helping to clear infections
- Calming inflammation in the respiratory system and other areas of the body
- Soothing sore muscles and joints
- Encouraging circulation
- Easing headaches (Try it in an inhaler for this.)
- Mental motivation
- Energy, focus, and optimism

EUCALYPTUS'S NONPROFIT ORGANIZATION: BREATHE BETTER INTERNATIONAL

Eucalyptus essential oil is on a mission to help the world breathe easier.

It's from Australia, but it's known internationally for its nonprofit organization called Breathe Better International, which plants trees to help improve air quality all over the world.

Eucalyptus has planted forests full of trees on almost every continent and has a franchise of tree nurseries so that people can bring small trees into their homes. Its organization doesn't only deal with eucalyptus trees. It works with the native plants of local areas to be sure it's respecting the natural ecosystem. Eucalyptus's organization has worked with citrus trees, conifers, and less well-known plants like Saro in Madagascar.

Breathe Better International also plants herbs, flowers, and spices that are known to offer respiratory benefits. Rosemary and cardamom are a few popular ones.

Once it started filling the world with more trees and plants, Eucalyptus realized there were plenty of other ways it could go about its mission. It created natural therapeutic products so it could improve people's health in a more direct way. All of its products are sustainably sourced from the forests it has planted around the world. It makes respiratory inhalers, diffuser blends, and body oils that help ease aches and pains during cold and flu season. Eucalyptus even created a line of natural cleaning products and air fresheners that fill your home with fresh energy.

Eucalyptus believes that taking the time to breathe deeply can help you connect with your vitality, your life, and yourself in important ways.

EUCALYPTUS'S SAFETY TIPS

Eucalyptus is a strong oil, and due to its chemical makeup, it is not my oil of choice for children under 10 years old, especially not in blends applied near their faces. For children under 10, I recommend using cedarwood instead. You can save eucalyptus for the bigger kids!

Before using eucalyptus essential oil for someone who suffers from asthma or another respiratory disorder, have them smell the lid of the oil's bottle first. If it makes their chest feel a little tight or constricted, use another oil for them. (Cedarwood is a good choice.) If it makes their chest feel more open, go ahead and see how a low dilution of eucalyptus makes them feel.

It is best stored away from homeopathic remedies.

Frankincense

Common name: Frankincense
Latin name: *Boswellia carterii*
Aroma: Fresh and "balsamic" (try smelling balsamic vinegar, then smell frankincense essential oil, and you'll detect the balsamic note). Soft, woody, and comforting.
Aromatic note: Middle-Top

FRANKINCENSE'S GIFTS

When the frankincense tree's trunk or branches are injured, the tree's resin comes out from within the tree to heal the wound. The essential oil is distilled from this resin. You can see this as frankincense's way of helping you draw on inner strength to stay healthy.

Frankincense is one of the best skin healers in the essential oil world, right up there with lavender and helichrysum. It calms inflammation and is known to have antioxidant and skin-healing properties. Long-term conditions like scars respond well to frankincense.

It offers protective effects to your respiratory system too. Frankincense can help reduce congestion, mucus, inflammation, and can even ease pain.

You can also use the essential oil or the raw resin as incense. This is one of frankincense's most ancient applications. It's been used for prayers, meditation, and rituals for thousands of years. A meditation body oil with a few drops of frankincense can help center your mind and nourish your skin at the same time. The raw resin makes a beautiful loose incense, and you can add your own ingredients to personalize it. Dried herbs, flowers, and drops of essential oil are a few good ideas.

Overall, frankincense offers a kind of healing that begins from within, affecting your heart and mind as well as your body. Use it in blends for:

- Daily skin care
- Rejuvenating damaged skin
- Soothing skin irritation
- Respiratory support
- Clearing mucus and congestion
- Helping to clear infections
- Calming inflammation
- Relieving headaches
- Blends for children
- Meditation and contemplation
- Feeling relaxed and uplifted

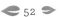

FRANKINCENSE'S MEDITATION CENTER

Frankincense runs a meditation center right in the middle of town.

Its doors are always open, and you're welcome to come anytime you would like to reconnect with yourself.

The entire building was handmade piece by piece, with love and attention to detail. It may seem a little exotic at first, but once you go, you'll feel right at home and you'll want to keep coming back. There's a main room where you can sit quietly and meditate with others, and a variety of smaller rooms where you can go if you'd like a little alone time.

Frankincense believes vibrant health comes from within, and there are many ways to access that. It teaches several kinds of yoga, tai chi, and meditation, and it has a class specifically focused on deep, healthy breathing. Frankincense makes all its own resin incenses, and always has a blend burning to help students deepen their breaths and calm their minds. It will be happy to give you a bag to take home!

Frankincense even offers relaxing muscle massages in private rooms with calm music, and you'll love the skin-soothing massage oil it uses.

Frankincense wants its meditation center to be a quiet spot in the middle of town and a peaceful spot in the middle of your day.

FRANKINCENSE'S SAFETY TIPS

Frankincense is a very safe oil. It's so gentle that it's one of my top picks for people with delicate systems, including children and the elderly.

A Frankincense Story

In Somaliland, the local frankincense harvesters leave their families for months at a time, climb into the mountains in their sandals, and hike through rugged terrain with small chisel knives and baskets.

When they get to the frankincense trees, they make "incisions" in the bark, and the trees produce a rich resin to heal the wound. The harvesters collect the resin when it dries.

My friend, the distiller Mahdi Ibrahim, is from Somaliland. He and his wife, Jamie, started an essential oil company called Boswellness in 2004 with the vision of providing pure Somaliland frankincense resins and oils to the public and getting the harvesters a fair price. They described their vision to a few friends, Casey Lyon and Bill Lanzetta, who saw that a real difference could be made and joined Boswellness to help.

There are no distilleries in Somaliland itself—water is extremely scarce in the region—so the four-person team at Boswellness imports the resins to their distillery in Vermont, USA. In fact, the process of essential oil distillation was unknown in Somaliland until very recently. When Mahdi told the Somaliland elders about his idea for a business partnership and showed them a little bottle of frankincense essential oil, they asked him, "How did you put our tree into this little bottle?"

To determine a fair price for the frankincense resin, Mahdi spoke to the harvesters themselves. When they told him what they thought would be fair, he doubled it. The business perspective in Somaliland—one which Mahdi and Boswellness share—is, "How can we collaborate for the community's well-being?" It's such a beautiful approach! The Boswellness team has already achieved funding for solar-powered wells and sanitation facilities in some of the Somaliland communities.

Mahdi, Jamie, Casey, and Billy have worked hard to become the first certified organic suppliers of frankincense resin and essential oil. In addition to empowering the people of Somaliland, they partner with Western researchers to learn more about the therapeutic properties of different frankincense species. I've been fortunate enough to visit Boswellness at their distillery in Vermont many times. I am impressed with the work they do and the products they create. Their commitment to education and providing the highest quality oils and hydrosols is an inspiration.

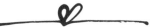

THE HEART OF AROMATHERAPY

Common name: Geranium
Latin name: *Pelargonium* × asperum
Aroma: Rosy and herbaceous, with hints of citrus
Aromatic note: Middle

GERANIUM'S RADIANCE

Geranium is a popular plant in gardens all around the world, and its familiar, rosy aroma inspires smiles and makes people feel good.

Geranium has a nourishing presence in skin-care blends of all kinds. It's good in blends for moisturizing dry skin, reducing acne, rejuvenating damaged skin, or for calming irritation that can lead to redness or swelling. It's also perfect for long-term skin conditions that cause irritation. Try pairing geranium with a resinous skin-loving oil, such as frankincense or myrrh, and blending it into your favorite unscented lotion or cream. It's helpful for reducing inflammation around scars.

Geranium is also good at easing pain—both physically and emotionally. It has a skill for calming inflammation and for offering emotional comfort at the same time. I especially like it in blends for chronically swollen joints and for swelling that can be traced to sluggish circulation in ankles or legs.

Like sweet orange, geranium is uplifting while also being soothing, so it's a good choice for blends to encourage you when you're feeling down. It's very gentle and is a good oil to turn to for long-term support, especially emotional support. You can also try it in a diffuser with other uplifting oils, such as the citruses (geranium smells wonderful with any citrus oil).

Geranium offers support for:

- Daily skin care
- Rejuvenating damaged skin
- Soothing skin irritation
- Calming inflammation
- Reducing swelling
- Feeling relaxed and uplifted

GERANIUM'S NATURAL SKIN-CARE SPA

Geranium has a real love of beauty.

It likes creating beautiful environments—with relaxing music, comfortable furniture, a welcoming aroma, and a little waterfall trickling in the corner. Environments like this make people feel good, and that's Geranium's goal.

It also knows that looking good and feeling good often go hand in hand. That's why it opened a skin-care spa.

Some people come to its spa to relax and rejuvenate. Geranium gives them aromatherapy baths, facial steams, and soap-free face washes, and whips up their favorite skin-loving blends on the spot.

Others come to ask Geranium about specific skin issues. It's an expert in keeping skin naturally clean and radiantly healthy. It also has special formulas for dry skin, and skin that's seen a lot of weather or has been damaged in some way.

For the really tough cases, Geranium consults with its friends Helichrysum, Frankincense, and Lavender, three other essential oils that have dedicated themselves to healing skin. Together they create oils and other products for reducing scars, soothing chronic irritation, and reducing inflammation.

Geranium is so popular because it always knows how to make people smile, and it's good at bringing out their natural beauty. You'll find your own reasons to love Geranium, and once you spend time with it, you'll be friends for life. Geranium treasures long-term friendships and will be there for you through thick and thin.

GERANIUM'S SAFETY TIPS

There are no specific safety concerns for geranium essential oil.

Common name: Ginger
Latin name: *Zingiber officinale*
Aroma: Spicy, warm, and radiant. Ginger's scent is powerful—a few drops go a long way!
Aromatic note: Middle

GINGER'S TALENTS

Ginger essential oil is wonderful for reducing pain. It has a warm, spicy effect that can be very soothing to areas that are chronically inflamed, tight, and constricted, which makes it a good addition to blends for sore muscles. I especially like ginger for pain that acts up in cold weather. It's a warming oil, so it's best used for conditions that feel cold. For example, chronically puffy joints that are cool to the touch as opposed to red and hot inflamed areas.

Some of the qualities that contribute to ginger's ability to ease pain have been researched, including its gifts for reducing inflammation, calming muscle spasms, and encouraging warmth and circulation.

These qualities make ginger a useful oil for blends that support the belly. It can help settle your stomach in a variety of circumstances—whether you've eaten something that doesn't agree with you, have nervous indigestion, are experiencing cramps, feel nauseous, or feel sick while you're traveling. It can even help with gas.

Ginger tends to dominate blends aromatically. If you're blending for a beautiful aroma, you may want to use only a few drops of ginger. This is also a good idea for topical blends, as too much ginger can irritate the skin. Be sure to balance it with a skin-nourishing oil, such as Roman chamomile.

Ginger is helpful for:

- Reducing swelling
- Soothing sore muscles and joints
- Calming muscle spasms and cramps
- Encouraging circulation and warmth
- Supporting digestion
- Easing nausea
- Energy, focus, and optimism

Essential Oil Profiles

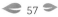

GINGER'S TRAVEL AND ADVENTURE AGENCY

Ginger is full of energy and spice, and loves to get out and see the world. It started a travel business to help others experience all the fun life has to offer!

Ginger will organize a trip that introduces you to new places, people, and foods. You'll travel by plane, train, boat, and car . . . and you'll never need to worry about travel sickness or nausea. Ginger always brings along essential oil blends to keep you comfortable.

One of the reasons it's so good at putting together adventures is that it seems to know exactly what you want to experience and takes you to all the right places. Do you need to breathe the freshest air? Ginger will take you on hikes through mountains and tropical rain forests. Want to explore natural healing traditions throughout the world? Ginger knows "medicine men" and healers in every country who can teach you about natural pain relief. Want to try new foods? Ginger will take you on a culinary tour of the globe, and it'll make sure your stomach is happy no matter what new foods you're trying.

Just be sure you're in good shape before signing on for one of Ginger's travel adventures. It loves keeping your energy up! It will take you out dancing late at night, and then take you on a long hike the next morning to show you the most inspiring landscapes.

GINGER'S SAFETY TIPS

Ginger essential oil can be skin-irritating for some people, as its spiciness can sometimes irritate mucous membranes. Blending it with other skin-nourishing oils can help sidestep that effect.

Common name: Gingergrass
Latin name: *Cymbopogon martinii* var. sofia
Aroma: Bright and herbal, layered with warm gingery, peppery, spicy notes. Sensual, complex. Hints of citrus (lemon) that are quite pronounced.
Aromatic note: Middle

GINGERGRASS'S FLAIR

Gingergrass is helpful for easing pain and getting your circulation going. It can be comforting in blends for sore muscles and stiff joints, whether the pain is acute or chronic. It has a fresh, herbal aroma that is both emotionally uplifting and relaxing. It's much easier to relax when you're feeling happy.

Gingergrass's circulatory qualities make it perfect for pain, inflammation, and swelling that flares up in cold weather. It blends well with other warming oils for this, such as cardamom. Be sure to blend the gingergrass and cardamom with a very skin-nourishing essential oil, such as geranium.

You'll find the way gingergrass gets your circulation going to be comforting and soothing, rather than too energizing. Its aroma can help to focus your mind and to ground you in the moment. Gingergrass is a good choice to help you stay relaxed throughout the day so you don't become stressed or tense. In this way, it can keep muscles happy and prevent pain from ever setting in.

Add gingergrass to your list of essential oils that help with respiratory issues. Just as its circulatory effects help it "get things moving," it gets things moving in your respiratory system too.

Gingergrass can help with:

- Respiratory support
- Reducing swelling
- Soothing sore muscles and joints
- Encouraging circulation
- Staying relaxed and happy all day long

GINGERGRASS'S DAILY YOGA AWARENESS CAMPAIGN

Gingergrass is from India, where it studied yoga all its life. It's older now, and it still practices yoga every day.

Gingergrass says that yoga makes it feel connected with life. In fact, yoga helps it feel so connected with life that it decided to do yoga every day in the middle of the town square.

At first people smiled at little old Gingergrass, stretching into seemingly impossible yoga poses while everyone walked by and went about their days. As day after day passed and Gingergrass continued to show up for yoga, people began to stop and watch. They admired Gingergrass's energy and vitality, and soon began asking it questions. Why was it doing so much yoga every day? Was it trying to raise awareness for some cause?

Gingergrass has a fun sense of humor and jokingly gave a different answer every day. All of its answers were true! Here are a few things Gingergrass said it's raising awareness for:

- Healthy muscles and joints, no matter your age
- Natural relief of pain
- The importance of deep, healthy, cleansing breath
- Keeping your body's circulation strong
- Staying relaxed in the middle of the flow of life

Gingergrass even smiled and said it was raising awareness for awareness. Some people found this a little confusing at first, but when they joined Gingergrass for yoga, they understood: working with Gingergrass made their minds feel more centered and present to the moment.

Now a small crowd gathers to do yoga with Gingergrass every day. Bergamot Mint is always there, and Lavender never misses a day. They say a little time with Gingergrass helps their entire day feel like it's flowing more smoothly.

GINGERGRASS'S SAFETY TIPS

Gingergrass can be sensitizing to skin if it is oxidized.

Common name: Helichrysum, Everlasting, and Immortelle
Latin name: *Helichrysum italicum*
Aroma: Rich, dense, and curry-like, with sweet almost fruity notes. Hints of honey and distinctly herbaceous.
Aromatic note: Middle

HELICHRYSUM'S BRILLIANCE

Helichrysum is a fantastic healer that can restore us from the inside out, and the outside in. It can help with bruises, cuts and scrapes, burns (especially sunburns), and bites and stings, and can reduce lingering effects of old wounds, such as scars.

In fact, maybe a list of skin issues that helichrysum *isn't* helpful for would be shorter than a list of what it *is* helpful for!

Helichrysum diffuses well, but is considered a "precious" oil. It's expensive due to the amount of labor that goes into hand-harvesting and distilling the very tiny flowers. Instead of diffusing it, I usually reserve it for skin applications so it can do its best work where it's most needed.

In small concentrations, I love helichrysum for everyday skin care. It earned its other names—"everlasting" and "immortelle"—because the tiny little yellow flowers never seem to lose their color or shape, even after the plant has been cut. It always looks vibrant and alive. It can share this skill with you and keep your skin healthy over time.

Helichrysum is an excellent choice for:

- Daily skin care
- Rejuvenating damaged skin
- Soothing skin irritation
- Calming inflammation
- Soothing burns
- Reducing scars
- Bruises, cuts, and scrapes
- Bug bites and stings
- Healing emotional wounds

RESTORE YOUR HEALTH AT HELICHRYSUM'S NATURAL WELLNESS CENTER

Helichrysum can't stand to see anybody hurt! When it was young, it employed the ever-popular "kiss it and make it better" technique.

Now that it's all grown up, it runs a natural wellness center. It doesn't want to be there for you only when you're injured and need help. It wants to help you preserve your health from day to day. It's a master of both preventive and restorative health care.

Visit Helichrysum's wellness center to restore your spirit after a long, difficult experience, or when you're going through a big life change. This is the place to reconnect with yourself and ask your heart what it needs to shine its brightest.

If something goes wrong—maybe you get an injury or illness—and you need a little more attention, Helichrysum will be at your bedside with its team of expert healers. They make their own healing products and practice natural therapies from around the world, and they'll sit with you until you're feeling better.

Then you can spend time in the wellness center's gardens, taking deep clear breaths of fresh air and admiring the flowers. Don't worry about the bees and bugs. Helichrysum knows how to handle stings, bites, and other surprise skin issues that pop up!

HELICHRYSUM'S SAFETY TIPS

Helichrysum is a very skin-nourishing and safe oil, but there's one consideration to keep in mind. It's not used on puncture wounds because helichrysum heals skin quite quickly. Punctures need to heal more slowly, from the inside out, so they don't get infected.

A Helichrysum Story

Helichrysum grows all over the island of Corsica, located off the coasts of Italy and France. It grows in the mountains, along the roadsides, in the fields, and can even be seen on the beaches popping up from the sand.

My friend Christina and I visited a lovely woman on Corsica, Michelle, who distills helichrysum essential oil. We took a small plane from Nice, France, to a tiny little island airport with a single airstrip, and rented a car from the one rental car company on offer. We had a general sense of the direction the distillery was in, which was good because there were no road signs! We made a few wrong turns and had to stop for directions several times. We laughed a lot and eventually found our way to the village where Michelle and her family work.

We had a delicious late night French dinner in the village, surrounded by old stone buildings with terra-cotta roofs, and the next morning we were up early with Michelle and her crew. They took us up a mountain where they had a permit to harvest wild helichrysum. We used hand sickles to cut the plants, filling basket after basket. I had never harvested helichrysum before, and it was a lot of work! We spent all day—eight hours—working with our hands, pausing only for a big picnic lunch and delicious afternoon tea.

After a full day of harvesting helichrysum, we had 66 pounds of flowering tops including leaves and flowers. We brought it all back down the mountain and distilled it, yielding 2.6 oz (about 78 ml) of essential oil. It really did take a *huge* amount of plant material to produce a little bit of oil!

We washed our faces with the helichrysum hydrosol, and Michelle told us a local story.

She said the island of Corsica has been fought over for centuries, and the land had seen a great deal of war. The locals believe that helichrysum grows all over the island to help heal the wounds of those wars—both physically and emotionally.

That's the perfect expression of helichrysum's personality as a dedicated healer.

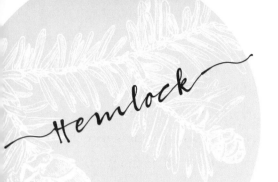

Common name: Hemlock, Canadian Hemlock, Spruce

Latin name: *Tsuga canadensis*

Aroma: Piney, fresh, and woodsy

Aromatic note: Top-Middle

HEMLOCK'S EXPERTISE

It's easy to confuse *Tsuga canadensis* with the poisonous plant that's also commonly called "hemlock," but they belong to entirely different genus and species. The toxic "hemlocks" are herbaceous members of the parsley family, while *Tsuga canadensis* is a conifer tree with a whole array of health-supporting properties.

Hemlock has been used for generations to boost immunity, calm inflammation, and support respiratory health. The Native Americans used hemlock branches in steam for sweat lodges. The steam would support their health and reduce infection.

You can get those same effects from hemlock essential oil by diffusing it or using it in an inhaler. Inhaling hemlock feels comforting when your body is clearing congestion, and it's so good at helping to reduce infections that it's a good choice for natural cleaning blends. Hemlock can also comfort spastic coughs.

It's an effective oil for pain relief, tension, and sore muscles. Try it in topical blends for cramps.

While hemlock can soothe muscles, it does so in a way that releases energy rather than relaxes it. Hemlock is a great essential oil for feeling vibrant and overcoming fatigue, especially during the long, dark months of the year. It blends well with black spruce.

Hemlock trees have a very long lifespan—some people estimate they can live over 800 years! Hemlock essential oil won't help you live quite that long, but it can certainly help you stay healthy and feel full of life.

Turn to hemlock for:

- Respiratory support
- Clearing mucus and congestion
- Easing sore throats and coughs
- Helping to clear infections
- Calming inflammation
- Soothing sore muscles
- Natural cleaning blends
- Calming muscle spasms and cramps
- Supporting overall immunity and vitality

HEMLOCK'S SCHOOL FOR "BUDDING" CONIFERS

Hemlock has lived a long time and has learned a lot about what it means to be a conifer. It opened a school in New England, where it teaches younger trees how to access their talents.

Hemlock's students have different goals. Some want to open massage practices, some want to make their own natural body products, and some simply want to learn how to care for others and be the best conifers they can be.

Black Spruce studied with Hemlock to learn how to help people feel vibrant and happy, especially during long, dark winter days that can drag their spirits down. Juniper studied with Hemlock to learn how to soothe muscle cramps. Piñon Pine went to Hemlock's school, and they increased each other's knowledge of ancient therapeutic techniques.

In Hemlock's classes, all the students call one another by their full Latin names. No common names allowed. This is because Hemlock has been confused for poisonous plants in the past, which made people afraid of it even though it's such a friendly old soul!

HEMLOCK'S SAFETY TIPS

Before using hemlock essential oil for someone who suffers from asthma or another respiratory disorder, have them smell the lid of the oil's bottle. If it makes their chest feel a little tight or constricted, use another oil for them. (Cedarwood is a good choice.) If it makes their chest feel more open, go ahead and see how a low dilution of hemlock makes them feel.

juniper

Common name: Juniper
Latin name: *Juniperus communis*
Aroma: Piney and fresh, with sharper resinous notes reminiscent of frankincense
Aromatic note: Top-Middle

JUNIPER'S GENIUS

Juniper is one of the oldest plants we know of to be used by humanity. The ancient Greeks and Romans loved burning juniper as incense, to repel bugs, and to cleanse the air in their homes. The Native Americans and Tibetans also used juniper for rituals and therapeutic purposes.

You can diffuse juniper essential oil to put a modern twist on those ancient uses. Try blending it with piñon pine and lemon in your diffuser. Not only does it create a fresh, foresty aroma in your home—it can help break up congestion. It can also have that effect in an aromatherapy inhaler (which is a convenient way to take juniper on the go with you) or a steam blend (which is comforting if you're clearing away sinus congestion or getting over a cold).

Juniper is also excellent at helping the body get through infections. You can use it topically for this purpose. Juniper works well in chest rubs and body butters, and even oils to soothe ear infections. It can help to soothe allover aches and pains during an illness too.

Juniper especially sparkles in blends for reducing swelling in joints, muscles, limbs, and connective tissues. When the area feels cool and swollen, juniper can introduce warmth and encourage circulation.

Emotionally, juniper inspires vitality and encouragement. It's as though juniper "gets things moving" in your body and your emotions at the same time.

Juniper essential oil can help you with:

- Respiratory support, especially for colds, flu, and congestion
- Helping to clear infections
- Reducing swelling
- Soothing sore muscles and joints
- Encouraging circulation and warmth (Try it for cold hands and feet!)
- Supporting overall energy and vitality

JUNIPER'S REJUVENATING JOINT MASSAGE

Juniper knew from the time it was young that it didn't want to go into the family business. Its family had been working wood with their hands for generations, and their hand-made furniture business had a reputation for lasting quality and comfort.

However, Juniper saw how working with their hands led to uncomfortable joint pain for a lot of its family members so it started learning massage techniques to help them feel better. After mastering massage, it started making its own pain relief gels, oils, and butters to enhance its work. Juniper's grandparents and great-grandparents especially love receiving massages. Their hands and feet always seem to feel cold and achy, but Juniper's TLC helps to clear that right up. They call Juniper "Junior," and say it is wise beyond its years. Grandpa Hemlock even got out of his rocking chair and did a dance after one of "Junior's" massages!

Juniper's family encouraged it to start another branch of the family business. Now it has a team of massage therapists working for it, and it sells its soothing products to clients. Juniper is always diffusing a welcoming, refreshing blend of conifer and citrus essential oils in its massage office. Simply waiting for your appointment can make you feel good!

When people first meet Juniper, they sometimes feel that it isn't taking their problems seriously—Juniper is upbeat and optimistic, even in the face of real discomfort and discouragement. That's Juniper's natural confidence coming through. It knows that it can help you feel better in no time.

JUNIPER'S SAFETY TIPS

Juniper can potentially irritate sensitive skin and can be sensitizing to skin if it is oxidized.

Essential Oil Profiles

A JUNIPER STORY

The country of Canada is rich with gorgeous conifer forests sweeping across huge areas of the landscape. The first time I visited my friend Lucie Mainguy, of Aliksir Distillery in Canada, I was truly inspired. It was easy to understand how such a place could be the source of many of my favorite conifer oils, and I was excited to meet this extraordinary woman and her family who work so hard to produce pine, spruce, and fir essential oils.

I had been in touch with Lucie for a long time, and I already loved Aliksir's essential oils (especially their balsam poplar and black spruce). When I actually saw the distillery, located on a small farm tucked away in a rural, forested area outside Quebec City, I fell in love with the entire operation.

Lucie started Aliksir Distillery with her husband in 1988, and it remains a small family business focused on working with naturally therapeutic plants and essential oils. She showed me her stills, two of which were built by her son, and told me about the process they use to create balsam poplar essential oil. It involves hand-harvesting twigs and buds from the trees in the spring, cutting the material into smaller pieces that are ready to go into the still, and then distilling for many hours on end. I finally understood the precious cost of this particular essential oil.

Aliksir also produces hydrosols. When I visited, Lucie shared a new product she'd been working on—Essential Waters. She uses a special proprietary technique to emulsify a plant's hydrosol and essential oil, combining their strengths into a product that's stronger than a hydrosol but still gentler than an essential oil. Her Essential Waters are all water-soluble, and she uses them like hydrosols. I was able to try her peppermint and cardamom Essential Waters, and loved their effects (and still do!).

Aliksir has grown a lot since their founding. They distill not only various conifer oils but a number of other plants, such as goldenrod and melissa. They sell their products in a little boutique store attached right to the distillery, and they import other essential oils from distillers around the world.

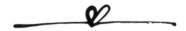

Common name: Kunzea
Latin name: *Kunzea ambigua*
Aroma: Medicinal, eucalyptus-like, a little spicy, and fresh
Aromatic note: Middle

KUNZEA'S MAGIC

Kunzea has a lot in common with eucalyptus and the conifer oils in that it's excellent for respiratory support, reducing infections, and soothing sore muscles. It combines the best of both worlds into a single oil.

Kunzea is from Australia, and like eucalyptus and rosalina (also from Australia), it's a strong oil for reducing inflammation and congestion. Its aroma has a medicinal note to it but is also comforting and soft. Blend kunzea with bright, penetrating oils like eucalyptus and rosemary ct. camphor, and it will help to soften the blend's sharp edges.

Kunzea's ability to calm inflammation means it's also useful for helping to ease different kinds of pain, such as headaches. If you experience sinus headaches, you can create a real "dream team" of essential oils with kunzea and a few of the conifers, such as hemlock and piñon pine. Use them in an inhaler to ease sinus congestion and headaches.

Whether it's in a topical blend or one for inhalation, kunzea can also soothe sore muscles. It smells so good paired with cedarwood in a restoring, revitalizing body oil.

It also has a reputation for repelling insects. In Australia, animals are known to curl up and sleep under kunzea trees because insects aren't fond of the aroma (although humans love it!). Try the essential oil in your own blends for discouraging bugs.

Use kunzea for:

- Respiratory support
- Clearing mucus and congestion
- Sinus headaches from allergies, colds, and flu
- Calming inflammation
- Soothing sore muscles
- Feeling relaxed and inspired
- Repelling insects

KUNZEA'S AROMATHERAPIST EXCHANGE PROGRAM

Kunzea is from Australia, and loves adventure and travel. During a trip to Canada, it fell in love with the beauty of the country's conifer forests.

Kunzea made friends in Canada who distill conifer essential oils and make their own aromatherapy products. Long talks over dinners showed everyone that although they came from different sides of the world, they had so much in common!

That's why Kunzea started the Aussie-Canadian Aromatherapist Exchange Program. It connects people who are passionate about essential oils in both countries so they can travel and stay with one another. Australian aromatherapists love staying with Canadian friends and learning about the amazing properties of conifer essential oils, like black spruce and hemlock.

Once they get back to Australia, they're happy to invite their new Canadian friends to come visit, and to take them on tours of eucalyptus, rosalina, kunzea, and more of Australia's unique plant life.

Kunzea's exchange program has made many new friendships possible. It has also resulted in some creative aromatherapy blends, as friends collaborate on recipes to combine Canadian conifers and Australian oils in fun, effective ways.

It's a simple truth that Kunzea still finds so profound—plants that come from different sides of the world can have a lot in common. The same goes for people!

KUNZEA'S SAFETY TIPS

Kunzea can be sensitizing to skin if it is oxidized. Although it is often used safely with children over five years old, kunzea does have some similarities to eucalyptus, so I use only 1 or 2 drops per 1 oz (30 ml) of carrier for kids' blends (and I often use cedarwood instead of kunzea).

Common name: Lavender
Latin name: *Lavandula angustifolia*
Aroma: Floral, fresh, sweet, woody, and herbal
Aromatic note: Middle-Top

LAVENDER'S SKILLS

Lavender is one of the most versatile, nourishing, and all-around supportive essential oils. I can't say it's good at everything, but it's good at *almost* everything!

Lavender really shines in blends for topical application and inhalation. You can use it for skin care, relaxation, respiratory support, and cleaning blends, especially paired with tea tree.

Making safe blends for children becomes easier with a bottle of lavender essential oil in your collection. It's gentle and versatile, and kids tend to love the aroma. Reach for lavender when you want to calm something down, such as a skin reaction, and offer emotional comfort. It helps kids (and adults) get to sleep.

Although it's very soft and gentle, lavender is also strong. It's a great addition to blends for reducing inflammation and helping skin heal. Lavender can help with acute pain, like a bug bite, and is nourishing enough for long-term use.

Lavender blends well with nearly all of the other essential oils in this book, and can substitute many of them in your recipes.

A short list of what lavender can help with includes:

- Daily skin care
- Soothing skin irritation and inflammation
- Respiratory support
- Soothing allergies and sinus congestion
- Helping to clear infections
- Soothing burns and reducing scars
- Bruises, cuts, bites, and stings
- Blends for children
- Natural cleaning blends
- Calming the nervous system to inspire deep relaxation and sleep
- Emotional balance and reassurance

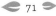

Essential Oil Profiles

LAVENDER IS A PARENT WHO WANTS TO CARE FOR YOUR WHOLE NEIGHBORHOOD!

Lavender essential oil has mastered so many arts that it could never have settled into a single profession. Instead, it uses all of its many talents in the most important job of all: being a parent!

Lavender is nurturing, supportive, and uplifting. It knows how to make people feel good, encourages them when they're stressed, and adds a touch of beauty everywhere it goes.

Lavender has a big purple house that all the parents in the community know and love. Its yard is always full of kids playing and having fun. If someone falls down, gets a bruise or a scrape, or gets stung or bit by a bug, Lavender takes out its homemade "first-aid kit" full of natural blends. It knows how to fix just about any little injury, including sprained muscles and twisted ankles.

Its yard is spacious, full of beautiful flowers and herbs, with plenty of trees that offer shade from the sun. It's the perfect place to stretch out in a hammock and take a nap.

Despite its home being a center of activity, Lavender keeps a very clean and tidy house, and makes all its own natural cleaning products. It won't hear of you helping to clean up after the kids! It wants you to relax and may even make you a comforting bath salt to use before bed.

LAVENDER'S SAFETY TIPS

Lavender is one of the safest and gentlest essential oils. The only safety tip is "don't leave home without it"!

A Lavender Story

The Lavender Way is a small-scale distiller on the island of Crete in Greece. They produce organic lavender essential oil, and other products made with lavender, such as potpourri sachets. I love their essential oil, and when I began talking with Gill and Derek, who started the Lavender Way, I fell in love with what they told me about their distillery. I wanted to see it all firsthand!

It was some time before I was able to take a trip to Crete, but when I finally arrived, the wait was worth it. Gill and Derek were just as wonderful in person as they'd been over e-mail. We shared a delicious lunch in the local village before they showed me around their farm and distillery, where they grow many different species of lavender and olive trees side by side, and where they have a gorgeous view of the brilliant blue Aegean Sea.

For Gill and Derek, the Lavender Way is not only the name of their business, it's a way of life. They are fully committed to cultivating their plants without the use of any chemicals and interacting with the plants and land using their hands as much as possible—that means no power tools and no tilling the land. They cultivate their plants in concentric circles so the plants can protect one another from pests. They do all their pruning by hand. It takes longer and the work is tougher, but they feel it helps create a stronger relationship between the people and the plants.

When I use Gill and Derek's lavender essential oil, it's as though the bottle in my hand is filled with the love they pour into their plants.

Common name: Lemon
Latin name: *Citrus limon*
Aroma: Bright, sharp, zesty, fresh, and lemony
Aromatic note: Top

LEMON'S BRILLIANCE

Lemon is one of my top choices for natural cleaning blends. You can use it in your kitchen and bathroom, and in natural, skin-nourishing hand cleansers. Its bright, sparkly top note complements most other oils used for cleaning. Try it with lime, peppermint, and lavender.

You can use lemon in blends that support your health too—especially respiratory health. As it helps to reduce infection and congestion, it also inspires you to feel happy and energized. Using an aromatherapy inhaler with lemon essential oil is an effective way to stay healthy and keep your heart lively throughout the day. It makes an excellent "travel buddy," especially when you're surrounded by other travelers and want to keep your immunity strong.

Lemon is phototoxic, so be sure to use less than 12 drops for every 1 oz (30 ml) of carrier oil. That said, it can help reduce pain, so try it in a blend for muscles and joints, especially if you'd like your blend to have a gentle cooling effect. Blend it with skin-nourishing oils, such as palmarosa.

Lemon is ideal for:

- Respiratory support
- Soothing allergies and sinus congestion
- Clearing mucus and congestion
- Helping to clear infections
- Reducing swelling
- Natural cleaning blends
- Feeling energized and inspired

LEMON'S BRIGHT LIFE AROMATHERAPY BAR

Lemon is passionate about helping people experience each day as a vibrant slice of life. It has fun doing this by running an essential oil blending bar.

Stop into Lemon's Bright Life Aromatherapy Bar to share fun stories with friends while making your own aromatherapy products. When you walk in, you'll immediately notice the fresh, fruity, uplifting aroma. The counters are stacked with natural, raw carrier oils and butters, and shelves of essential oils line the walls. There are cabinets full of sparkling empty bottles and jars for you to work with.

You can make one of the blends on Lemon's "menu"—a list of the most popular aromatherapy products people like to make—or get creative and make your own unique blend. Lemon is always happy to offer ideas and help you personalize its popular recipes.

When Lemon isn't measuring carrier butters, blending essential oils, or making people laugh, it's cleaning. It is dedicated to keeping a pristine kitchen! It wouldn't want any cleaning chemicals around its organic products, so it makes its own cleaners. Lemon likes everything to be as natural as possible!

LEMON'S SAFETY TIPS

Lemon is a phototoxic essential oil. Please read more about phototoxicity on **page 17**.

You can sidestep lemon's phototoxicity by sticking to less than 12 drops per 1 oz (30 ml) of carrier oil.

Citrus trees can be heavily sprayed with herbicides and pesticides. I recommend buying lemon essential oil produced from organically grown fruit.

Lemon can be sensitizing to skin if it is oxidized.

Common name: Lime
Latin name: *Citrus aurantifolia*
Aroma: Bright, zesty, and sparkly, like a freshly cut lime
Aromatic note: Top

LIME'S FLAIR

Lime is the perfect essential oil for mornings, after work, or anytime you might need an infusion of energy. Its scent is radiant and inviting—it can help you greet the day with an open heart!

Lime is a brilliant addition to blends for cleaning, and works on surfaces and in diffusers to keep your environment sparkling and healthy. Try blending it with tea tree. They can both reduce infection, and lime's sparkly aroma balances tea tree's more medicinal scent. I always use distilled lime, because cold-pressed lime is phototoxic and distilled lime is not.

Lime is so good for reducing infections, and you can also use it in blends to ward off a cold or flu.

One of the brightest ways lime shines is in belly blends, such as creams for nausea and digestion. Blend lime into an oil to rub on your low back and belly after a big meal, or into a cream to soothe stomach cramps. If you're not sure what's upsetting your stomach but are definitely sure you want to feel better, lime can help.

Lime is useful for:

- Respiratory support
- Soothing allergies and sinus congestion
- Clearing mucus and congestion
- Supporting digestion
- Easing nausea
- Natural cleaning blends
- Feeling energized and uplifted

DISTILLED LIME HOSTS THE MOST FUN OUTDOOR DINNER PARTIES!

Lime essential oil loves connecting with friends, and is always hosting dinner parties!

It has a backyard picnic table in a small garden shaded by several lime trees, jasmine vines, and rose bushes, and the air is fresh and fragrant. Lime serves fresh-squeezed juice and homemade salsa, but be sure to wash your hands before you take a seat (with Lime's handmade foam soap)! Lime has a reputation for cleanliness.

The other citruses love to come to Lime's dinner parties. The meals are always healthy, mouthwatering dishes that Lime learned while it was traveling in the islands. If your stomach doesn't always digest new foods easily, Lime has you covered. Everyone gets a jar of soothing belly cream as a party favor!

After dinner, Lime will turn on fun salsa music and have everyone dancing around the yard. Don't worry about cleaning up the postmeal mess—Lime loves to clean! It likes to make all its own cleaning products.

Make yourself at home in Lime's home, and spend some time breathing in the fresh air and feeling good!

LIME'S SAFETY TIPS

Cold-pressed lime essential oil is phototoxic, but *distilled* lime is not phototoxic. The Latin names are the same (*Citrus aurantifolia*) so be sure to check how the oil was obtained when you're purchasing it. Please read more about phototoxicity on **page 17**.

Citrus trees can be heavily sprayed with herbicides and pesticides. I recommend buying lime essential oil produced from organically grown fruit.

Lime can be sensitizing to skin if it is oxidized.

myrrh

Common name: Myrrh

Latin name: *Commiphora myrrha*

Aroma: Resinous, warm, and spicy. When it's "young," the oil has a sharp, medicinal element, which seems to soften as the oil ages.

Aromatic note: Base

MYRRH'S GIFTS

Myrrh resin has been used throughout history as incense for rituals, and to purify the space in temples. It's still used in this way today, as myrrh can help people release stress and come to a place of trust in their hearts.

Myrrh can nourish skin, calm inflammation and redness, and soothe irritation. It has been used in blends for beautiful skin since the time of the ancient Egyptians, and is still cited for its skin-nourishing benefits in hot, dry climates. It's excellent in salves for dry, cracked skin, and gentle enough for everyday use in body creams and oils. It's also strong enough for more acute issues, like bug bites and blisters.

Myrrh is a wonderful choice for supporting open breathing. Try it in a blend to help break up mucus. Its soothing effect can help you feel comforted while your body clears congestion. The essential oil can clog in a diffuser, but that's not an issue in an inhaler.

It's also good for topical blends. Myrrh's skin-nourishing abilities make it perfect for body oils to ease muscle aches during a cold or flu. If your blends include oils that might irritate skin, such as juniper, adding a few drops of myrrh can reduce that potential for irritation.

Myrrh is perfect for aches and pains that aren't associated with a cold too. Try it in blends for joints that feel cool and swollen for its comforting, warming effect.

Myrrh is excellent for:

- Daily skin care
- Rejuvenating damaged skin
- Soothing skin irritation
- Respiratory support
- Clearing mucus and congestion
- Calming inflammation
- Bug bites and stings
- Warming
- Meditation and contemplation
- Emotional peace and tranquility

MYRRH'S ROADSIDE SHRINES

Myrrh likes to create what it calls "roadside shrines"—little pockets of calm, beauty, and sacred space in the middle of everyday life.

When you see rocks stacked atop one another in an almost "magical" balancing act, that's Myrrh's work.

When you see inspiring chalk drawings on the sides of buildings, that's Myrrh in action too.

Myrrh likes to spell inspiring words with rocks in the middle of the desert so you can see them when you drive through, and draw hearts in the sand on the beach. It's very fulfilled when it can help people stop, center themselves, and feel good.

After several years of traveling as a "roadside shriner," Myrrh realized it could give people little moments of sacred space in more personal ways too. It created its own line of skin-care and body products to sell at street fairs and farmers' markets. Its booth is the one on the corner, burning resin incense that brings in customers. Stop by Myrrh's booth, and it will give you a hand massage with "Nourished from Within" Body Oil (a recipe it made with its friend Frankincense), or make you a "Seriously Soothing" Chest Rub (created with its friend Saro) for that cough you can't shake. It has an intuition for knowing what your body needs to get in touch with its own peace.

Myrrh even passes out free aromatherapy inhalers to help people breathe deeply and feel peaceful all day. It never runs out of ideas for how to make "moments of magic."

MYRRH'S SAFETY TIPS

Myrrh is a safe essential oil overall. However, it is on the pregnancy avoid list in Robert Tisserand and Rodney Young's book, *Essential Oil Safety*.

myrtle

Common name: Myrtle, Green Myrtle, Common Myrtle, True Myrtle
Latin name: *Myrtus communis*
Aroma: Soft and fresh, with strong lemony notes. A camphoraceous accent with sweet floral notes that prevent it from smelling too medicinal.
Aromatic note: Top

MYRTLE'S TALENTS

Open a bottle of myrtle essential oil, and you'll immediately know it's an amazing choice for respiratory support. It has a fresh, sweet aroma, and one whiff of it can make you feel like you're already breathing more evenly and deeply. There is a soft, gentle quality to myrtle that encourages you to relax into deep, open breathing.

If you have a cold that comes along with a sore throat and cough, myrtle can help. It can also support your body as it clears out thick mucus. It combines a lot of respiratory relief in a single essential oil.

A body oil with myrtle can help to calm inflammation, and can feel so good if you've got the flu and all the physical aches and pains that come with it. Myrtle also offers a lot of relief for muscle spasms and tension. Try blending myrtle with black spruce, spike lavender, and ginger to bring out its ability to offer allover relief.

Myrtle is also useful for easing upset stomachs and supporting digestion. Try it in an inhaler to reduce nausea or if you eat something that doesn't agree with you. A nausea inhaler with myrtle can also help you breathe more deeply and feel healthier overall.

Myrtle is gentle and strong, and can have an impressive effect in blends for:

- Respiratory support
- Soothing allergies and sinus congestion
- Clearing mucus and congestion
- Easing sore throats and coughs
- Helping to clear infections

- Calming inflammation
- Soothing sore muscles
- Supporting digestion
- Easing nausea
- Feeling relaxed and uplifted

MYRTLE'S HEALING WATERS HOT SPRINGS

When Myrtle opened its little rustic hot springs resort, it knew it had found the perfect way to support people's health.

The hot springs naturally bubble up out of the ground, and Myrtle has planted the area with aromatic flowers, trees, and herbs that help people breathe more deeply. You'll love being in the hot springs while tiny rosemary flowers, kunzea blossoms, and eucalyptus leaves fall in and float around you. They create an aromatic steam coming up from the warm water that can help to open your sinuses and release congestion. It's been known to soothe spastic coughs.

The warm water helps your muscles release tension too. In the rare case that a customer still feels a little tense after a soak in the hot springs, Myrtle has a wonderful massage therapist on hand who will be happy to help.

Myrtle goes out of its way to make sure its customers feel happy and healthy. It serves a light, easy-to-digest dinner every evening at an outdoor table in the fresh air. When it's time to leave, you'll receive a complimentary body lotion, inhaler, and essential oil steam blend, so you can take the soothing effects of Myrtle's hot springs with you after you leave.

MYRTLE'S SAFETY TIPS

Before using myrtle essential oil for someone who suffers from asthma or another respiratory disorder, have them smell the lid of the oil's bottle first. If it makes their chest feel a little tight or constricted, use another oil for them. (Cedarwood is a good choice.) If it makes their chest feel more open, go ahead and see how a low dilution of myrtle makes them feel.

Based on the chemistry, Robert Tisserand and Rodney Young, authors of *Essential Oil Safety*, suggest staying under a 2% dilution when blending with myrtle for topical use.

A Myrtle Story

Tucked away in the mountains of Crete, Greece, off a one-lane road (you'll have to pull to the side if you meet someone coming in the opposite direction!), is a little shop and café called Wild Herbs of Crete.

The stone building with its assortment of wood and stone tables out front seems to come out of nowhere when you turn a corner in the road, and the colorful hand-painted wooden signs add to the welcoming atmosphere.

Even if we hadn't meant to go there, Christina and I would not have been able to resist stopping in for a cup of tea.

Wild Herbs of Crete is run by Babis and Janina, who started it in 1994. They create and sell a variety of essential oils and herbal products, including myrtle essential oil, handmade soap, and dried herbs. They have no farm at Wild Herbs of Crete, but harvest all their herbs from wild plants growing in abundant populations in rural areas. Babis and Janina never kill a plant to obtain its oil and don't employ workers who might not share their values for the plants' integrity.

Their kitchen was full of essential oils, fresh and dried herbs (including drying bundles hanging upside down from the ceiling), hydrosols, other natural and local products, and plenty of sunlight and fresh mountain air. Janina's cooking was delicious, and we were fortunate to taste a lot of it as we stayed in her guest room for two days.

Babis and Janina's first still was a traditional Cretan model from 1924. They have larger equipment these days but no plans to expand their business into a "big operation." Their goal is to remain a family business, staying small enough so that they can continue working with the local plant populations with no danger of overharvesting.

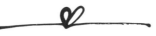

Common name: Neroli
Latin name: *Citrus aurantium* var. amara
Aroma: Soft, floral, and citrusy. Deeply calming, yet uplifting.
Aromatic note: Middle

NEROLI'S RADIANCE

The bitter orange tree that produces neroli is one of the few known plants that actually produces three different essential oils. Neroli essential oil comes from the flowers, petitgrain essential oil comes from the leaves and twigs, and bitter orange essential oil comes from the rind of the fruit.

Neroli's enchanting aroma makes it a popular essential oil for natural perfumes. The scent of neroli has been shown to have a deeply soothing effect on the nervous system, which means that neroli perfumes not only make you smell amazing, but help you stay happy and centered. It blends well with a number of other perfume-perfect oils, such as patchouli and opopanax.

Neroli is a very emotionally reassuring essential oil. Keep your neroli blends with you when you're feeling anxious or going through times of change or loss, to help comfort and reassure your heart.

A neroli perfume, body oil, or body butter seems to offer skin the same balance and harmony that it inspires emotionally. It helps calm inflammation, reduce redness, and support skin's radiance. You can also try it in a massage oil to bring these effects to sore muscles. Neroli is often used to ease muscle tension and cramps.

Neroli is a precious essential oil with a "low yield," meaning that it takes a lot of blossoms to create a single drop. It costs more than most essential oils, but it's quite strong and a few drops will do.

Neroli is wonderful for:

- Daily skin care
- Rejuvenating damaged skin
- Soothing skin irritation
- Calming inflammation
- Soothing sore muscles
- Natural perfumes
- Emotional comfort
- Feeling centered and relaxed

NEROLI'S NATURAL PERFUMES AND POTIONS SHOP

Neroli runs a natural perfume shop in Tunisia. Its store has earned a reputation for "magic potions," since each of its perfumes has a deeply inspiring, almost transformative effect on the wearer.

It crafts perfumes designed to make people smile, relax them into a sweet sleep, or help them fall in love! You can buy a bottle of perfume, or ask Neroli to blend your favorite scent into a skin-nourishing body butter or oil. It loves providing what you need. And if you're not sure what you need, Neroli has a blend for that too. Try the "My Body Is a Temple" Body Oil, which can help you feel grounded and centered, and help you get in touch with your own inner guidance.

Neroli loves to travel and makes friends from all over the world, who make sure to stop by the perfume shop when they pass through Tunisia. They're always introducing Neroli to new scents, and giving it fresh ideas for "magical" perfumes that affect people's lives.

Neroli loves to host "perfume parties" once a month, when it keeps its shop open late and invites everyone in town to come and make their own natural perfume blend. There is a minor cover charge, but nobody minds because they all come away with a perfume that suits their personality, brings out their best, and supports them through whatever is going on.

NEROLI'S SAFETY TIPS

Neroli is a very safe essential oil. However, using too many drops can become overwhelming and cause a headache, so sticking with a few drops is a good idea.

Common name: Opopanax, Sweet Myrrh
Latin name: *Commiphora guidotti*
Aroma: Resinous, with deep, warm, sweet, and spicy notes. Hints of black licorice.
Aromatic note: Base

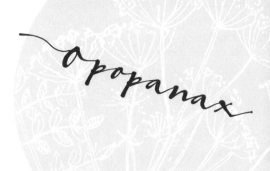

OPOPANAX'S EXPERTISE

Opopanax resin has always been highly valued as incense for use in meditation, rituals, and contemplation. Both the raw resin and the essential oil are used in this way today. You can make a loose incense blend or a meditation oil and sit quietly with opopanax, letting the aroma wrap around you, comfort you, and encourage your mind to release worries. This is one of those essential oils that helps people feel grounded and present, and realize the peace that each moment offers.

Opopanax has been used since ancient times for healing skin. Oils distilled from resins tend to be strongly supportive in this way, reducing inflammation and rejuvenating skin's resilience. Opopanax is no exception.

The deep, sweet aroma of opopanax can act as a base for a wide variety of scents, including florals, citruses, woods, and other base notes. It has been a popular ingredient in perfumes throughout history, and when historical sources refer to "myrrh," they often mean opopanax.

Opopanax perfumes and skin care often accomplish the same things—nourishing you while helping you smell good.

Opopanax is a great choice for:

- Daily skin care
- Rejuvenating damaged skin
- Soothing skin irritation
- Reducing inflammation
- Natural perfumes
- Meditation and contemplation

OPOPANAX THE ARCHAEOLOGIST

Opopanax believes the past is very present, and is full of gifts for us today.

That's why it works as an archaeologist. It spends a lot of time in the Middle East, and especially Egypt. Using all the latest technology and approaching its dig sites with the utmost respect, it uncovers ancient monuments, temples, statues, and sometimes finds scrolls full of writing.

Its team often spends days on dig sites, and Opopanax always makes sure everyone is well nourished. It provides plenty of water, and makes sure the entire team has shade and skin care to protect them in the heat. If anyone gets bitten by a bug or develops a blister from working with hand tools, Opopanax is right there to soothe them. At the end of every long, dusty day, everyone gets to freshen up with Opopanax's handmade soaps and deodorants. Resting peacefully under the stars is never a problem—Opopanax burns incense to help its team feel meditative and relaxed.

Opopanax's favorite findings are ancient jars full of resins and oils, or recipes for incense or natural perfumes. Its team loves identifying the aromatic materials that have been preserved for thousands of years and recreating recipes that haven't been made in centuries.

Opopanax believes when you spend time with yourself and "dig deep," you can find your own wisdom and peace.

OPOPANAX'S SAFETY TIPS

Opopanax is known to be safe and healing, but according to Robert Tisserand and Rodney Young, authors of *Essential Oil Safety*, it could potentially cause some skin irritation. Blend it at a low dilution of about 1 percent.

Common name: Sweet Orange
(also called Orange)
Latin name: *Citrus sinensis*
Aroma: Warm, bright, radiant, and citrusy
Aromatic note: Top

ORANGE'S SWEETNESS

Sweet orange is a powerful and versatile oil, yet it's so gentle that it's perfect in blends for children—which is great, because kids love the juicy scent of orange!

One of sweet orange's most impressive effects is supporting happy, comfortable bellies. It's perfect for indigestion, nausea, and stomach tension. Since it's gentle for skin, it works well in topical blends, such as a belly butter with Roman chamomile, as well as in blends for inhalation. Aromatherapy inhalers with sweet orange are reliable for keeping "quick comfort" on hand, and kids can use them all by themselves.

Another benefit of inhaling sweet orange is that it can help support clear breathing. The familiar aroma is fortifying as your body clears infections.

One reason it supports deep breathing is because it helps calm inflammation and tension. Tension seems to dissipate in the presence of sweet orange, whether it's physical or emotional tension. Its comforting scent can set your mind at ease as well as your body, and it's so bright and sunny that it's easy to feel optimistic when you're using sweet orange.

Sweet orange creates comfort and health all around. It can even help clean up your environment since it's good for reducing infections.

Use sweet orange for:
- Respiratory support
- Soothing allergies and sinus congestion
- Clearing mucus and congestion
- Helping to clear infections
- Calming inflammation
- Supporting digestion
- Easing nausea
- Blends for children
- Natural cleaning blends
- Feeling relaxed, restored, and uplifted

Essential Oil Profiles

VISIT SWEET ORANGE'S ORCHARD RETREAT

Sweet Orange is the friend you've known for years who never lets you down—familiar, warm, and always there when you need a bit of comfort.

Visit Sweet Orange at its home in a warm, sunny orchard. You're always welcome, and no worries are allowed there! Sweet Orange will help you let go of anxiety, stress, and frustration. It will massage the tension out of your muscles, give you space to breathe, and remind you of the beauty in your life until you're feeling healthy, revitalized, and optimistic.

No one goes hungry in Sweet Orange's house. Its home is full of good, nourishing foods that can restore your health, and of course they're easy to digest! After a delicious meal, Sweet Orange will clean everything up itself (it makes all its own natural cleaning blends), and then pour you a warm bath. You'll have no trouble drifting off to sleep after that! Relaxation comes easily in Sweet Orange's warm glow.

In fact, spending time with Sweet Orange makes everything feel like it's flowing more easily—feelings, thoughts, goals, and health.

SWEET ORANGE'S SAFETY TIPS

Sweet orange essential oil is not phototoxic, but it can be sensitizing to skin if it's oxidized.

Citrus trees can be heavily sprayed with pesticides, which come through the cold-pressing process and are found in the essential oil. I recommend buying sweet orange oil produced from organically grown fruit.

GC/MS Reports

GC/MS stands for "Gas Chromatography/Mass Spectrometry." A GC/MS report provides a breakdown of the natural chemical components in an oil. GC/MS can help you confirm that the oil is pure, identify some potential therapeutic properties of the oil, and point toward any safety considerations to keep in mind.

Fortunately, my early education included studying GC/MS and how to read the reports. When I was first buying essential oils, I often bought through aromatherapy companies, not directly from distillers. This meant the essential oil went from the distiller to at least one distributor (maybe two) and then to the aromatherapy company I purchased from.

One year, I bought a 32 oz (960 ml) bottle of frankincense from an essential oil company I trusted and liked. When it arrived, I had it tested with GC/MS. When the test results came back, I was shocked—the essential oil was adulterated. It was only 2 percent true frankincense! It was 98 percent synthetic!

The oil smelled wonderful because the adulterant was odorless. If not for the GC/MS report, I would never have known it was adulterated.

My shock jump-started my dedicated and passionate journey to find essential oil distillers whom I could buy from directly.

Buying directly from distillers is a great way to reduce the chance of buying adulterated essential oils because the distillers are not known to adulterate their oils. It's generally the middle people, the distributors, who "cut" essential oils with cheaper essential oils or synthetic substances for financial gain. This is a widespread practice that motivates me to work with and support small-scale distillers around the world. These distillers are hard-working organic farmers and are proud of the oils they distill.

I recommend buying essential oils from a company that buys directly from the distillers.

Many essential oil companies test their essential oils with GC/MS. It's too expensive for individual buyers to have their oils tested, but the bigger, more established aromatherapy companies can afford to do it. I appreciate when an essential oil company tests its oils and is willing to provide the GC/MS report to customers if asked. The quality of your therapeutic blends depends on the quality of your oils. Seeing the long list of chemical components present in the oil, and the percentages they show up in, may not mean much to the beginning aromatherapist, but it can be very useful for a certified aromatherapist.

When you're deciding where to buy your essential oils, feel free to ask companies whether they test their oils with GC/MS and if they make the reports available to customers. Here are a few questions that can help you make your decision:

- Are all of your essential oils tested with GC/MS technology?

- Can you provide the GC/MS report for the oil that I buy?

- What is the oil's country of origin, and the year and season the oil was produced?

- Are the oils imported directly from the distillers who produce them?

- Which of your current essential oils are organic or "unsprayed" (grown without pesticides and herbicides, but not necessarily certified organic)?

If the company you're thinking of purchasing from doesn't do GC/MS tests on every batch of their essential oils, that doesn't mean their oils are adulterated. Some of the smaller essential oil companies simply cannot afford to test their oils. The last three questions on the list can still tell you a lot about the oils and about how the company considers their quality control.

Common name: Palmarosa

Latin name: *Cymbopogon martinii* var. motia

Aroma: Rosy and herbal, with a lemony, woody undertone. Pleasantly floral, lighter and less dominant than some of the heavier floral essential oils such as rose or ylang ylang.

Aromatic note: Middle

PALMAROSA'S STRENGTHS

Palmarosa essential oil is a wonderful choice for skin-care blends. It can nourish your skin on a day-to-day basis, and it's very supportive when skin needs a little more care and attention. Palmarosa can help reduce redness, irritation, and inflammation.

Palmarosa also has gentle cooling effects and can feel refreshing in blends for areas that are a little red and overheated, or blends that you like to use on hot summer days. A blend with palmarosa can be applied to the back of your neck as a perfume that can also help cool you down. This is an effective way to soothe a headache too.

These cooling, inflammation-calming effects are great for reducing swelling, especially swelling in joints that feels warm. It complements juniper, lemon, and German chamomile in blends for easing pain.

Like many floral essential oils, palmarosa has a comforting effect on our emotions. It is helpful for emotional stress that tends to translate into physical tension in the body. Its aroma is reassuring and peaceful, with a sweetness that seems to radiate through the heart and mind. Try it in an allergy-calming linen spray.

You can count on palmarosa in blends for:

- Daily skin care
- Rejuvenating damaged skin
- Soothing skin irritation
- Respiratory support
- Reducing swelling
- Soothing sore muscles and joints
- Emotional comfort and relaxation

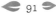

PALMAROSA'S PLANT CONSERVATORY AND RESEARCH CENTER

Palmarosa knew from a young age that it wanted to spend its life learning everything it could about how to care for skin . . . and then putting that knowledge into practice.

That's why it runs a research center in India, studying skin and creating nourishing body products. Stepping into its laboratory is like walking into a botanic conservatory, with plants from all around the world growing everywhere you look.

Palmarosa is always researching both ancient and new plant therapies from around the world. It loves to travel and talk with traditional healers, learning about how they do their work, and it often brings back new plants and essential oils to study at its conservatory.

Needless to say, Palmarosa has collected a lot of plant wisdom from around the world. Despite all its research on natural healing, Palmarosa still likes to remind people of the body's innate wisdom—especially as it shows up in their skin. Our skin itches when something irritates us, gets chills before we come down with a cold, gets goose bumps when we're nervous or afraid, and shivers when we're excited about something. Palmarosa likes to say, "Your skin will tell you what's going on."

PALMAROSA'S SAFETY TIPS

Palmarosa is a very safe essential oil.

Common name: Palo Santo
Latin name: *Bursera graveolens*
Aroma: Woody, smoky, sweet, and spicy,
 with subtle hints of citrus
Aromatic note: Middle-Base

PALO SANTO'S MAGIC

"Palo santo" means "holy wood." The tree grows in Ecuador and the Galapagos Islands. In Ecuador, the indigenous peoples have long used palo santo for health, rituals, purification, protection, and meditation.

Obtaining palo santo essential oil is a unique process. The oil is present only two years after the tree has died naturally. The oil doesn't form in trees that are harvested before they naturally fall. During these years, the tree's resin permeates the wood. After that time, the wood chips can be steam distilled to produce the oil.

Palo santo is useful in blends to help your body recover from a cold or flu. Since it's deeply skin-nourishing, you can use it in blends for topical application as well as inhalation. A moisturizing body oil with palo santo can help you rest when you're sick and can soothe achy muscles since the essential oil is good for reducing inflammation. The aroma is woody and reassuring, which is always welcome when you're feeling under the weather.

Palo santo wood is often used as incense, so if you'd prefer to save the essential oil for topical blends, you can still inhale palo santo by adding the essential oil or wood chips to an incense blend. It has the added benefit of helping to center and focus your mind. The wood is also burned to keep away insects—a nice perk that palo santo offers! You can get this effect more directly by blending the essential oil into a lotion to keep bugs away from your skin.

Use palo santo for:

- Daily skin care
- Rejuvenating damaged skin
- Soothing skin irritation
- Respiratory support
- Soothing allergies and sinus congestion
- Calming inflammation
- Repelling insects
- Natural perfumes
- Meditation and contemplation
- Feeling centered and focused

PROTECT INDIGENOUS PEOPLES WITH PALO SANTO

Palo Santo grew up in Ecuador, raised near a community of the Native indigenous people who have lived in the rain forests for generations. It grew up learning natural healing techniques and ancient wisdom.

Later on, Palo Santo traveled the world and saw that much of the wisdom it was raised with had been lost. So it decided to give back in the best way it knew how: it started an organization to protect indigenous peoples around the world, and to educate others about the wisdom of their lifestyles and traditions.

Its favorite way to do this is making modern products based on ancient recipes. It makes body oils that nourish skin, and restore skin when it's irritated and inflamed. Palo Santo's perfumes and incense are said to be "protective," as they help calm people's emotions.

Palo Santo uses all-natural ingredients, sustainably sourced from forests and wild places all around the world. It loves using traditional production techniques, and includes photographs of the people who make its ingredients with each of its orders so customers can really get to know who they're supporting with their purchase.

Palo Santo loves to help people feel connected to one another, and to nourish them on the inside as well as the outside.

PALO SANTO'S SAFETY TIPS

In their book *Essential Oil Safety*, Robert Tisserand and Rodney Young suggest using Palo Santo topically at no more than a 3% dilution.

Common name: Patchouli
Latin name: *Pogostemon cablin*
Aroma: Heavy, rich, earthy, and sweet. Multifaceted and complementary with many other oils.
Aromatic note: Base

PATCHOULI'S PASSION

Patchouli essential oil is known for many qualities, but some of its most famous uses are for skin care and relaxation.

It's nourishing and restorative, and encourages any inflamed, irritated areas to calm down. Since patchouli is a heavier essential oil that nourishes skin, it's a good choice for topical blends, such as body butters or moisturizing oils, but it's thick enough that it doesn't always diffuse well. A few drops can provide your blends with a grounding base note that complements scents such as German chamomile, palmarosa, and neroli.

Patchouli oil has a long history of being used in perfumes and natural pest repellents, and it works well as a natural deodorant. It's gentle enough for sensitive areas of skin such as under your arms, although you may need to apply natural deodorants more often than others.

Patchouli is known to deeply relax the nervous system. This is an essential oil to use when it's time to lie back and fall asleep, or when you want to sit quietly in meditation and let your mind and body harmonize in a peaceful way.

The essential oil ages very well—so much so that "vintage" or "aged" patchouli is a popular variation of the oil.

Reach for patchouli for:

- Natural perfumes and deodorants
- Daily skin care
- Rejuvenating damaged skin
- Soothing skin irritation
- Calming inflammation
- Bug bites and stings
- Repelling insects
- Meditation and contemplation
- Feeling deeply relaxed and peaceful

TUNE IN TO PATCHOULI'S PEACE-OUT RADIO STATION

Patchouli's motto is "Peace out," and it wants to spread its message of peace far and wide. It also loves bringing people together and having a good time, so it runs a radio station that plays nothing but music from the 1960s!

Everyone who works at Patchouli's radio station is chilled out, relaxed, and happy. They also get a lot done. Patchouli is always organizing ways to make people feel good, and its station has become a center where the community is all welcome. They have "dance hour" every day at noon, and "drumming and singing hour" every evening. People love to come relax in its "urban hot springs"—a bunch of small, heated pools and hot tubs that mimic Patchouli's favorite natural hot springs and that make people's skin feel good.

Patchouli even has a 24-hour "nap room," with dim lights, relaxing music, and incense. Drop in and curl up in a hammock or bean bag chair and get a little rest!

Patchouli has a lot of personality, and it gets along with nearly everyone. It has a laid-back attitude that reminds its friends not to take anything so seriously that it spoils their good mood. At parties, Patchouli's simple presence can have such a calming effect on everyone in the room.

PATCHOULI'S SAFETY TIPS

Patchouli is generally a very safe essential oil. It's generally considered safe during pregnancy; however, it is cautioned against using while breast-feeding as it could pass into breast milk.

A Patchouli Story

The Seychelles used to be one of the main producers of patchouli essential oil. Patchouli grew everywhere on the islands, and you could even find it springing up along the sides of the roads. However, it was so plentiful that the locals considered it a weed, and many patchouli plants were pulled up so the land could be developed. Now there's a lot less patchouli in the Seychelles.

In 2014, I participated in a two-week perfumery course in the Seychelles run by Isabelle Gellé from the Perfumery Art School. As a small archipelago in the Indian Ocean, the climate of the Seychelles is very tropical. The water was clear and turquoise, banana trees and other tropical plants lined the roads, and jasmine and bougainvillea grew in cultivated areas. What a paradise!

The only essential oil distiller in the Seychelles islands is a man named Mustafa Bristol. He made it his personal mission to grow as much patchouli as he could and to provide the local organic farmers with the plants so they could reintroduce it to the islands. He had already started the nursery and showed me about 100 gorgeous, healthy plants. He loves raising his plants organically and producing the highest quality essential oils. He even built his own stills!

Following my visit, Mustafa built a facility to produce organic coconut oil. Coconut oil production is another practice the Seychelles have been known for throughout history, and Mustafa is taking part in that tradition.

Aromahead Institute and Aromatics International, a company focused on importing essential oils and carriers directly from distillers, have both contributed to Mustafa's costs to support his coconut oil and patchouli projects. It's fulfilling to be able to support small-scale distillers and farmers like Mustafa who are doing such important work!

Mustafa also distills lemongrass, cinnamon, and a few other essential oils, but patchouli and coconut oil remain his most passionate projects. It was such a privilege to see him work, and I can't wait to return to the Seychelles and see his progress.

Essential Oil Profiles

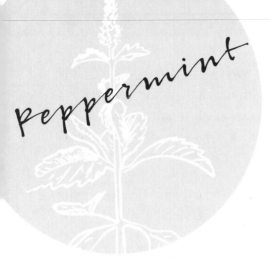

peppermint

Common name: Peppermint
Latin name: *Mentha × piperita*
Aroma: Minty, fresh, bright, penetrating, and oh-so-sweet!
Aromatic note: Middle-Top

PEPPERMINT'S BRILLIANCE

Peppermint essential oil can claim the spotlight in your blends. A few drops are usually enough to balance even strong aromas, such as Roman chamomile.

One of my favorite ways to use peppermint is for stomach troubles, such as nausea and indigestion. Use your peppermint blends before or after a big meal, or both. An inhaler with peppermint can actually help ease digestion and relieve a headache at the same time.

Inhaling peppermint is refreshing, and can help clear congestion and "open your senses." It's known for reducing infection too. Reach for peppermint if you have a cold or flu, or if you're making natural cleaning products.

In topical blends, peppermint has an "icy-hot" cooling sensation—a hallmark sign that it's helping to reduce inflammation and get circulation going. That sensation also makes peppermint helpful for sore muscles and joints.

This is a potent, penetrating essential oil that can feel like a blast of fresh air and a burst of fresh energy.

Use peppermint for:

- Respiratory support
- Clearing mucus and congestion
- Reducing swelling
- Soothing sore muscles and joints
- Helping to clear infections
- Supporting digestion

- Easing nausea
- Encouraging circulation
- An "icy-hot" effect
- Natural cleaning blends
- Uplifting and energizing yourself
- Focusing and sharpening your mind

GO OUT ON THE TOWN WITH PEPPERMINT

Peppermint is ultracool, and always leaves a good impression on new friends. You'll be hard pressed to find someone who doesn't adore Peppermint after getting to know it! It loves to relieve stress and have fun, and it brings a breath of fresh air everywhere it goes.

Peppermint loves to take friends out on the town for dinner and dancing. You'll enjoy a meal full of delicious foods, and Peppermint will be there to help you digest in comfort so you're not too full to dance.

Peppermint doesn't want anything to get in the way of your good time. If you're feeling a little under the weather, Peppermint will make a congestion clearing blend to help you feel better. If you have a headache, Peppermint will be right there to ease your head and massage your sore muscles. It will even put a soft, lavender-scented eye pillow over your eyes so menthol fumes don't get to them.

Your friend Peppermint may keep you up late, but it will also help you get up bright and early the next morning. An A.M. visit from Peppermint can help you to get a fresh start to your day. Peppermint is simply a reliable friend—there for you anytime you need to feel uplifted.

PEPPERMINT'S SAFETY TIPS

Peppermint creates a soothing "icy-hot" feeling when applied to skin, but applying too much can take it over into "burning hot" and cause irritation. Avoid using peppermint near the eyes, as the fumes can cause irritation. Peppermint can also irritate skin in a bath. Occasionally, people experience skin or mucous membrane irritation when using peppermint.

For children, dilute it at a maximum of 0.5%.

Peppermint is best stored away from homeopathic remedies.

Common name: Piñon Pine
Latin name: *Pinus edulis*
Aroma: A familiar evergreen aroma, with a sweet freshness and hints of citrus that places it among the top notes
Aromatic note: Top

PIÑON PINE'S GENIUS

Piñon pine also goes by the names "pinion," "pin-yon," and "pinon." In southwestern American states, where it's known for producing pine nuts, it's often spelled "piñon." It has such wonderful therapeutic properties that the Native Americans used it in many natural remedies and rituals for supporting well-being and reducing infections.

You can turn to piñon pine essential oil for the same things. If you've ever walked through a forest of conifer trees and noticed how fresh the air was, you can get an idea of how piñon pine can help your body clear congestion.

If you suffer from allergies and don't like to think of walking through that conifer forest, piñon pine can still help. Take along an inhaler with piñon pine and use it to help continually calm reactions to allergens, including inflammation and congestion. You can also diffuse the essential oil to cleanse the air and create an inspiring atmosphere.

As it's useful for helping to calm inflammation, try piñon pine in blends to ease pain—especially sinus headaches, or sore muscles and joints. An inhaler with piñon pine can help to release tension, and you can also make topical blends to massage it into sore muscles and joints.

Piñon pine essential oil is also a perfect ingredient for alcohol-free hand cleansers.

Use piñon pine essential oil for:

- Respiratory support, including allergies
- Soothing allergies and sinus congestion
- Clearing mucus and congestion
- Easing sore throats and coughs
- Helping to clear infections

- Calming inflammation
- Relieving headaches
- Feeling inspired, uplifted, and motivated

PIÑON PINE'S SOUTHWEST OUTDOOR RESTAURANT

Piñon Pine has lived all over the American Southwest, and loves the food from that region so much that it decided to open a restaurant . . . with a unique twist.

To get there, go on a little hike into the forest. Piñon Pine's restaurant is a simple open-air structure with a few outdoor cooking ovens and picnic tables all around. The menu changes from day to day, but Piñon Pine always sprinkles a handful of pine nuts over every dish.

Piñon Pine makes sure its guests are comfortable. If your skin starts feeling dry or irritated in the southwestern air, Piñon Pine will make you a nourishing body butter. It also makes massage oil. Some guests feel a little sore after hiking to its restaurant, so Piñon Pine's friends offer massages while it prepares dinner. If you're concerned about eating outdoors because of allergies, don't worry—Piñon Pine has aromatherapy inhalers on hand, and burns its handmade incense to keep away bugs.

Its restaurant may be outdoors, but Piñon Pine is not okay with uncleanliness. A little dirt is one thing, but it keeps all its cooking surfaces sparkling clean, and is always reaching for its bottle of alcohol-free hand cleanser.

PIÑON PINE'S SAFETY TIPS

Before using piñon pine essential oil for someone who suffers from asthma or another respiratory disorder, have them smell the lid of the oil's bottle. If it makes their chest feel a little tight or constricted, use another oil for them. (Cedarwood is a good choice.) If it makes their chest feel more open, go ahead and see how a low dilution of piñon pine makes them feel.

Rosalina

Common name: Rosalina
Latin name: *Melaleuca ericifolia*
Aroma: Soft and floral, with a fresh medicinal note. A combination of lavender and tea tree aromas.
Aromatic note: Top

ROSALINA'S BEAUTY

Rosalina comes from Australia, where it's often grown near beehives for honey production. Just like lavender, bees love rosalina.

Rosalina is distilled to produce a charming, delicately scented essential oil. Its aroma is floral—but not *heavily* floral. It's also medicinal—but not *heavily* medicinal. Rosalina is known as "lavender tea tree," and its scent combines the best of both.

Rosalina is a good choice when you want the cleansing, therapeutic action of tea tree, but feel tea tree may be too strong. Try it in foam soaps, hand cleansers, dish soaps, and bath salts. Rosalina is strong enough to be effective in such cleansing blends. It's an excellent choice to fortify you against infection and help you stay healthy.

It can also help you breathe deeply, especially when you're recovering from an infection and feeling stuffed up with congestion. Rosalina works well in diffusers, and you can use it day or night. It has a very relaxing effect and is able to soothe and uplift you, like lavender.

You can use rosalina for:

- Respiratory support
- Soothing allergies and sinus congestion
- Clearing mucus and congestion
- Easing sore throats and coughs
- Helping to clear infections
- Calming inflammation
- Natural cleaning blends
- Feeling relaxed and uplifted

ROSALINA'S BEEKEEPING AND HONEY COMPANY

Rosalina lives in Australia, where it grows aromatic, flowering gardens, and keeps beehives to make its own honey.

Rosalina started selling honey at farmers' markets for fun. Word of mouth got around quickly! Soon local grocery stores asked to stock Rosalina's honey, and it set up a website in response to popular demand.

Rosalina also began making therapeutic products from its plants. It quietly brought its hand cleansers, diffuser blends, inhalers, and bath salts to the farmers' market, and was so pleased when its products started selling right away.

People like to hang out at Rosalina's booth because everything there smells good. It's always diffusing an essential oil blend that helps people breathe easily. It even gives away natural cleansers to keep people's hands clean.

Despite its recent success, Rosalina remains very humble. It doesn't advertise, and if you go looking for its gardens, you'll see a simple handmade sign pointing you down a dirt road. Rosalina will be happy to take you on a tour of the gardens, and will let you pick out a free jar of honey and your favorite therapeutic product to take home.

ROSALINA'S SAFETY TIPS

Before using rosalina essential oil for someone who suffers from asthma or another respiratory disorder, have them smell the lid of the oil's bottle. If it makes their chest feel a little tight or constricted, use another oil for them. (Cedarwood is a good choice.) If it makes their chest feel more open, go ahead and see how a low dilution of rosalina makes them feel.

Rosalina is not known to be especially skin-irritating, but due to its chemical makeup, it's still a good idea to blend it with other skin-supportive oils. Although it is often used safely with children over five years old, rosalina does have some similarities to eucalyptus, so use only 1 or 2 drops per 1 ounce (30 milliliters) of carrier for children's blends (and I often use cedarwood instead of rosalina).

Rose

Common name: Rose
Latin name: *Rosa × damascena*
Aroma: Very rich, heavy, sweet, and floral
Aromatic note: Middle-Base

ROSE'S RADIANCE

Rose's reputation usually precedes it. Everyone is familiar with its sweet aroma and the beauty of its flowers. However, not everyone is familiar with its many uses in aromatherapy. Some of its more popular properties have to do with supporting healthy, beautiful skin.

Rose is especially helpful in blends for mature or very dry skin. Try a gentle exfoliating scrub with white clay and a single drop of rose oil, and follow it up with a face spritz made of rose hydrosol. Rose hydrosol blends well with vetiver hydrosol—try combining them in your face spritz.

As it brings out natural beauty, rose can also nourish self-love. Using inhalers or perfume oil made with rose can help you express the best parts of yourself and appreciate your beauty from day to day. Rose is also known to soothe emotional wounds. It inspires love and lifts the spirit, while also having a calming effect on the nervous system. If you're feeling low-spirited before bedtime, try a rose perfume oil to comfort and relax yourself as you go to sleep.

The comfort it offers your heart is reflected in the gentle pain relieving effect rose has in blends for sore muscles, joints, or other physical discomfort. Blend it into a tension-soothing bath salt with Roman chamomile and frankincense.

Rose is a strongly fragrant oil, and too much can easily overwhelm the aroma of a blend. Fortunately, a single drop is often all you need. Rose otto is obtained via steam distillation, and rose absolute (which smells just as sweet but is more affordable) is obtained by a process called "solvent extraction."

Rose is good for:

- Daily skin care
- Rejuvenating damaged skin
- Soothing skin irritation
- Calming inflammation and redness
- Toning and freshening skin
- Natural perfumes
- Comforting and uplifting the heart
- Feeling relaxed and optimistic

ROSE'S LOVE AND RELATIONSHIPS ADVICE COLUMN

Rose sees the world through "rose-tinted glasses." Everywhere it goes, it's always helping people recognize the beauty all around them and bringing out the love in their hearts.

It runs an advice column for love and relationships so it can help people far and wide. Rose's column is popular because it always offers practical solutions and sound advice people can put into practice right away. It loves to ask, "What does your heart want to do today?"—an empowering question that helps people put love into practice.

Rose has advice on . . .

- Easing pain: "Take special care of yourself if you're injured. It's okay to rest."
- Feeling more beautiful: "Beauty is natural! Use your favorite natural skin care, eat healthy food, exercise, and make sure you laugh every day."
- Practicing self-love: "Every day is another chance for you to be your most authentic self."
- Navigating change: "Make choices that are grounded in love."
- Insecurity and fear: "Do everything from a place of love, and you can feel confident."

Rose's family has a long history of working in the perfume industry and still loves to make natural perfumes and body-care products. Every day, Rose sends a gift of natural perfumes and products to someone who reads its column. Gifts are always accompanied by big bouquets of roses.

ROSE'S SAFETY TIPS

Rose is very strong, and just one drop goes a long way. In their book *Essential Oil Safety*, Robert Tisserand and Rodney Young suggest using rose otto at no more than a 0.6% dilution.

A ROSE STORY

Imagine having lunch in a garden in France, near a field full of 5,000 rose bushes in full bloom. The aroma of the roses fills the air, and the beautiful pink blossoms on the vibrant green bushes seem to embrace you on all sides as you indulge in fresh, local French bread, cheeses, olives, and lavender cookies.

That was exactly the scene my friend Rhiannon and I found ourselves in when we went to visit her friends at the distillery *Verdon Roses et Arômes* in France.

The distillers at *Verdon Roses et Arômes* are a husband and wife team named Jacky and Evelyne, and they harvest all their roses by hand with the workers on their farm. They have to harvest about 50 rose blossoms to get a single drop of rose essential oil. When you tip a bottle of rose essential oil to get out one drop, imagine four dozen roses coming out of the bottle!

There can be anywhere from about 500 to 900 drops of essential oil in a 1 oz (30 ml) bottle. This number varies based on the oil, the size of the orifice reducer, and the size of the drop. For this example, let's go with 600 drops. Remember, it takes about 50 roses to produce one drop. That means our 1 oz (30 ml) bottle with 600 drops has about 30,000 rose blossoms in it.

Jacky and Evelyne run a certified organic farm. They deeply respect the environment and the plants they care for, growing only species that are adapted to their specific area of the country. In addition to several species of roses, they grow and distill cornflowers, helichrysum, lavender, wild carrot, and a few other organic plants.

Verdon Roses et Arômes sells their hydrosols and essential oils, and they create their own line of skin-care products. Everything is of the highest quality, and their work continues to amaze and humble me.

Common name: Rosemary
Latin name: *Rosmarinus officinalis* ct. camphor
Aroma: Strong fresh, woody, herbal, and camphoraceous
Aromatic note: Top-Middle

ROSEMARY'S TALENTS

There are several chemotypes of rosemary, and different components are prominent in different chemotypes. The camphor chemotype is known for its energizing effects, respiratory support, and the way it can ease muscle aches and pains.

Rosemary ct. camphor is a wonderful essential oil to use in the morning, when it can get your energy flowing and help your mind feel more focused and clear. It diffuses well, so try a few drops in your diffuser as you go through your morning routine. You can also use it in an inhaler to help clear "brain fog" at work or during study time.

Using rosemary ct. camphor in a diffuser or inhaler is also an effective way to experience its respiratory benefits. It has anti-inflammatory properties that can be soothing during a cold or if you have allergies. Simply smelling the essential oil and feeling the way it opens up the breath can give you a good idea of the way it helps the body clear mucus. Its infection-reducing talents can support the body too.

Rosemary is also a perfect oil to use in blends that help calm inflammation and encourage circulation. Use it in a joint gel to reduce pain and swelling, or in a headache relief oil.

Overall, rosemary has a very uplifting effect. Reach for it when you want to get your blood pumping, your thoughts focused, and your energy flowing.

Rosemary is good for:

- Respiratory support
- Soothing allergies and sinus congestion
- Clearing mucus and congestion
- Reducing swelling
- Soothing sore muscles
- Encouraging circulation
- Relieving headaches
- Feeling energized
- Mental focus and clarity

ROSEMARY'S PEAK PERFORMANCE CENTER

Rosemary loves to see people perform at their best.

It feels happy to see its friends do well at work, ace a test, give an inspiring performance, run a fast race, and show the world what they're capable of.

It wants to empower everyone to do their best, so it started a community center where people can get into physical, mental, and emotional shape.

What's holding you back from doing your best? Rosemary wants to help in any way it can. If you're feeling sluggish, Rosemary will infuse you with motivation and inspiration. If you want to get your circulation moving, Rosemary will show you its exercise area. There are lots of classes to join and team sports to play. Then if your muscles are sore from exercising too hard, it has a team of massage therapists who can help work out your aches and pains. If you're feeling under the weather, spend time in its steam room to decongest. If you can't concentrate, Rosemary will give you peace and quiet, and help you focus so you feel productive.

Rosemary has gone out of its way to cover every base when it comes to helping you access your full potential.

ROSEMARY'S SAFETY TIPS

Rosemary is a "stimulating" essential oil, so I like to use it in blends for the morning and daytime, as opposed to before bed.

Rosemary ct. camphor is a strong oil (similar to eucalyptus) and is also not my oil of choice for children under 10 years old, especially not in blends applied near their face. Rather than rosemary, I often use orange, basil ct. linalool, and yuzu for kids between 5 and 10.

CHEMOTYPES:
SAME GENUS, SAME SPECIES, DIFFERENT ESSENTIAL OILS

Can two rosemary plants (both *Rosmarinus officinalis*) growing in two different places produce two different essential oils?

Yes!

This is part of the brilliance of plants. Sometimes, two plants of the exact same genus and species (in this case, *Rosmarinus officinalis*) can grow in two different geographical areas, and they can produce two different essential oils. The plants' genus and species are exactly the same, but the essential oils they create have different chemical components, aromas, and uses. These different oils are called "chemotypes," or "chemical types," and are shown with a "ct." in the essential oil's Latin name, as in "*Rosmarinus officinalis* ct. camphor."

Thyme is another good example. *Thymus vulgaris* ct. thymol is a wonderful oil for reducing infection, but it can irritate skin. *Thymus vulgaris* ct. linalool is also good at reducing infection, but is very gentle on skin—so much so that it's always my thyme oil of choice for kids' blends. You can see the genus and species are the same; it's only the chemotype that's different. You can also see why it's important to know the chemotype you're blending with, so you can make blends that are safe and effective.

Despite all our knowledge about the plant world, science is still uncertain about why only certain plants produce chemotypes. Thyme, basil, and rosemary are a few plants that produce chemotypes. These three plants have a genetic predisposition toward producing different chemotypes when planted in different environmental situations. However, not all aromatic plants behave this way. Sweet orange, for example, doesn't produce chemotypes. From country to country and from batch to batch, we can trust that different bottles of sweet orange essential oil will have pretty much the same chemical components and the same effects. The aroma can vary to some degree, but the overall chemistry is very similar.

You can think of chemotypes like identical twins that have different personalities. They look similar, but they like to do different things.

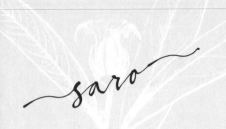

Common name: Saro
Latin name: *Cinnamosma fragrans*
Aroma: Warm, radiant, and camphoraceous, reminiscent of soft eucalyptus
Aromatic note: Middle-Top

SARO'S FLAIR

Saro essential oil offers a good alternative if you're looking for the effects of tea tree or eucalyptus, but want a softer camphoraceous aroma. Saro has a warmth to it that can be comforting when you need a little support to feel healthy, and it especially shines in blends for respiratory health and sore muscles.

Saro helps the body calm inflammation and clear infections, whether it's inhaled or used in topical blends. A combination of congestion, a headache, and sore muscles can be uncomfortable and keep you awake if you're exhausted, and saro can help on all those counts. It blends well with black spruce for this. It's relaxing enough to use in blends to help you fall asleep. You can use it in diffuser blends and linen sprays.

Saro also blends well with oils distilled from resins, such as myrrh and frankincense. This works out perfectly, because myrrh and frankincense offer a lot of protection for skin while complementing saro's ability to help reduce congestion and infections. They're also very emotionally relaxing.

You can even add saro to your natural cleaning blends if you prefer it over tea tree.

Reach for saro for:

- Respiratory support
- Soothing allergies and sinus congestion
- Clearing mucus and congestion
- Easing sore throats and coughs
- Helping to clear infections
- Calming inflammation
- Natural cleaning blends
- Feeling relaxed and uplifted

SARO'S "SPACE TO BREATHE" INTERNATIONAL AROMATHERAPY CO-OP

Saro lives in Madagascar, a country with some of the most unique plant and animal species in the world. It has traveled a lot and made friends in different countries, but it could never live anywhere other than its hometown.

So Saro came up with a way to "think globally, and act locally." It started an international aromatherapy co-op right there in Madagascar! Saro's co-op sells handmade organic products from all around the world. It has an exquisite respiratory body oil made by friends who distill conifer essential oils in Canada, and an aromatherapist in Morocco sends a pain relief blend that's very popular. The entire co-op always smells amazing because Saro loves to burn frankincense from its friends in Somaliland, and to diffuse essential oils to help its customers breathe easily.

All of Saro's aromatherapists find it refreshing that they have a place to sell their most unique creations. They say it's like having "space to breathe."

SARO'S SAFETY TIPS

Before using saro essential oil for someone who suffers from asthma or another respiratory disorder, have them smell the lid of the oil's bottle first. If it makes their chest feel a little tight or constricted, use another oil for them. (Cedarwood is a good choice.) If it makes their chest feel more open, go ahead and see how a low dilution of saro makes them feel.

Saro is a strong oil (similar to eucalyptus) and is not my oil of choice for children under 10 years old, especially not in blends applied near their faces. You can save saro for the bigger kids!

spike lavender

Common name: Spike Lavender
Latin name: _Lavandula latifolia_
Aroma: Floral, herbal, and fresh. It smells similar to true lavender, but with a sharper camphoraceous note that may remind you of rosemary ct. camphor or eucalyptus.
Aromatic note: Middle

SPIKE LAVENDER'S EXPERTISE

Spike lavender essential oil is nourishing to skin, just like true lavender. It's more energizing than true lavender though, so instead of helping you feel relaxed, it can help you feel more motivated. It also has some properties similar to eucalyptus, being wonderful for respiratory support and soothing sore muscles. Spike lavender is a useful essential oil for daytime, when you may want to take care of your muscles but don't actually have time to kick back and relax.

You can use spike lavender in a muscle oil to soothe painful tension, cramps, or strains after a strenuous activity, such as working out. A blend like this can also be helpful to massage your muscles with _before_ a workout to help get your circulation going and prevent issues like cramps. You'll notice it lends a slight cooling effect to topical blends.

Spike lavender also works well in inhalers. It's often used for reducing inflammation, and breathing spike lavender in can feel soothing if you have a cold.

True to its energizing nature, spike lavender is known to help people's minds feel more awake and focused. It complements rosemary ct. camphor very well—try them together in an inhaler to ease headaches and deepen concentration.

You can use spike lavender for:

- Respiratory support
- Soothing allergies and sinus congestion
- Clearing mucus and congestion
- Easing sore throats and coughs
- Helping to clear infections

- Calming inflammation
- Soothing sore muscles and joints
- Encouraging circulation
- Feeling motivated and energized

SPIKE LAVENDER'S SPORTS MASSAGE

Did you pull a muscle on your morning jog?

Hike a little too far yesterday?

Push your body too hard while playing a game with friends?

Spike Lavender is waiting on the sidelines to help you feel better and get back into the game. It's a sports massage therapist, which means it specializes in easing muscle strains, sprains, tension, inflammation, and other injuries that might develop while you're having fun.

Spike Lavender studied anatomy and physiology, and then traveled the world learning different massage techniques. On its travels, it met many natural healers who helped expand its understanding of pain relief.

Spike Lavender makes its own therapeutic products, such as muscle oil to prepare for a workout, inhalers to help athletes breathe deeply and reduce headaches, blends for focused concentration, and shower gels to help people feel clean and refreshed after a game.

You can think of Spike Lavender as true Lavender's more active, energetic cousin. True Lavender's mothering nature makes it good at nourishing, nurturing, and comforting you through life's stresses. Spike Lavender has the same comforting, nurturing personality, but with a "kick" that encourages you to get back out there and keep going. It loves giving pregame pep talks to make you feel empowered and congratulating you so you keep feeling good after you're done playing.

SPIKE LAVENDER'S SAFETY TIPS

Spike lavender can be energizing, so you may want to stick with it for daytime blends. Due to its chemical makeup, it's not my favorite oil for children under 10 years old. I recommend either using a few drops per 1 oz (30 ml) of carrier oil, or using Roman chamomile and true lavender instead.

spikenard

Common name: Spikenard
Latin name: *Nardostachys jatamansi*
Aroma: Heavy, earthy, and sweet, with warm hints of wood
Aromatic note: Base

SPIKENARD'S MAGIC

Spikenard oil comes primarily from India and Nepal, where it grows high in the Himalayas. It's been used for thousands of years in spiritual contexts such as rituals, prayer, meditation, and in temples and incense.

It's a deeply fragrant essential oil, with a sweet earthy scent that made it a popular ingredient in perfumes throughout the ancient world. Perfume oils with spikenard were often saved for special occasions, such as weddings and other ceremonies.

Spikenard's aroma is known to have a calming effect on the nervous system, which explains its use in meditation blends meant to center the mind and settle the emotions.

There is a deeply comforting aspect to this essential oil, which shows in its ability to reduce inflammation and help muscles relax. It's also a good addition to blends for nausea, digestion, and belly pain. Try blending a few drops of spikenard into a belly butter with sweet orange, Roman chamomile, and ginger.

Spikenard is a heavier essential oil, so I tend not to use it in my diffuser. However, it's right at home in body oils and butters, incense, and inhalers.

Reach for spikenard essential oil for:

- Calming inflammation
- Supporting digestion
- Easing nausea
- Natural perfumes
- Meditation and reflection
- Calming your nervous system
- Feeling relaxed and uplifted

SPIKENARD'S ANCIENT TEMPLE TOURS AND RETREATS

Spikenard essential oil is the most popular tour guide in India and Nepal, where it leads people on walking tours of ancient temples.

Far from just leading you around and explaining the history of each temple, Spikenard treats its tours as miniretreats. Plan to spend a few days hiking around the local area, sampling Indian and Nepali cuisine, and meditating in ancient temples. Spikenard will teach you to use the local plants to make your own modern version of ancient incense blends. It always brings along frankincense and opopanax resins for you to blend with.

Spikenard knows all that hiking can leave you a little sore. As you get quiet and reconnect with yourself, Spikenard will come around and massage your shoulders or sore muscles. It sees releasing physical tension and emotional tension as going hand in hand.

Treat Spikenard's "temple tour" as your time to reconnect with yourself. You'll spend time:

- Making incense to burn while you meditate, reflect, or journal
- Blending natural perfumes and body products that make you smell wonderful
- Gathering local plants that have traditionally been used for reducing inflammation and supporting health
- Eating delicious, healthy foods that your belly has no trouble digesting despite their exotic, spicy kick!

Spikenard sees our inner and outer worlds as connected and believes that well-being in one can reflect in the other. It believes there's a place within you that is always at peace, and that you can connect with this place by spending reflective time in the natural world. It calls this process "grounding" and likes to say "grounding is the first step toward soaring."

SPIKENARD'S SAFETY TIPS

Spikenard is a very safe and calming essential oil. Like sandalwood and rosewood, spikenard is now an endangered species, so I use this essential oil sparingly.

Tea Tree

Common name: Tea Tree
Latin name: _Melaleuca alternifolia_
Aroma: Fresh, herbal, and medicinal. Sharp and clean.
Aromatic note: Top-Middle

TEA TREE'S SKILLS

Tea tree's most popular uses revolve around different ways to clean things up, from your environment to your body (or your "in-vironment").

There aren't many natural substances that can reduce infection with the potency that tea tree can. It's one of my favorite choices for natural cleaning blends. I love it in surface cleaners, kitchen soaps, and blends to reduce the possibility of mold growth.

Tea tree diffuses very well and helps cleanse the air, so it's an excellent choice if someone in the house is sick and you'd like to prevent illness from spreading. Inhaling tea tree is a great way to reduce inflammation and get some relief from congestion.

You can also add it to an inhaler or do a steam with a _single_ drop of tea tree in a bowl of hot steamy water.

Tea tree is strong and gentle enough to cleanse your skin. You can use it in natural foam soaps, or alcohol-free hand cleansers to take with you and use wherever you are.

Tea tree is excellent for:

- Daily skin care
- Respiratory support
- Soothing allergies and sinus congestion
- Clearing mucus and congestion
- Easing sore throats and coughs
- Helping to clear infections
- Calming inflammation
- Natural cleaning blends
- Energy, focus, and optimism

TEA TREE'S NATURAL CLEANING BUSINESS

Tea Tree's home is always spic-and-span and ready for guests, but be prepared. If you visit, you'll be given a spray bottle and sponge and put to work cleaning. Tea Tree has high standards so don't let it catch you sitting around doing nothing when there's work to be done. Don't forget to take your shoes off at the door!

Tea Tree essential oil's motto is "clean = healthy = happy."

It admires what bleach can do, but prefers a natural approach. So it started its own natural cleaning business. Tea Tree's mission is to clean every home, office, massage room, and yoga studio—without relying on toxic chemicals.

It has a "dream team" of natural cleaners on its crew, and it always checks their work with a white glove. The dream team includes the citruses, conifers, and Lavender. (It's a good thing Lavender's on the crew! Lavender helps Tea Tree relax its uptight ways without relaxing its standards.)

Tea Tree's mission doesn't stop with external environments. It also goes after infections that make their way into your body, giving your inner environment the same white glove treatment it gives its cleaning crew.

It loves clearing away inflammation and congestion; it thinks mucus is "messy" and has no patience for it. Since it's good at cleaning up messes that can cause us discomfort, Tea Tree has also gotten a reputation for pain relief.

TEA TREE'S SAFETY TIPS

Tea tree essential oil can occasionally cause a skin-sensitization reaction.

Essential Oil Profiles

A Tea Tree Story

In 2013, my travel buddy Christina and I visited Clive and Jessica, my dear friends in South Africa who distill essential oils.

Clive's business is called Tuebes, and his daughter, Jessica, runs an offshoot of it focused exclusively on organic essential oils, carriers, and other natural products. The offshoot is called Scatters Oils.

Scatters supports small-scale farmers and essential oil distillers all over Africa. The farmers and distillers dedicate their time and attention to growing their plants and creating high-quality essential oils. They don't often have the resources to market or export those oils. That's where Jessica and Clive come in! Scatters helps these farmers get their essential oils to people all around the world who love them, and in the process, it supports rural communities.

On this particular trip, Jess and Clive took us to see citrus essential oil production on the border of Zimbabwe in the Limpopo region. The trees were a deep shade of green, abundant with bright citrus fruits. The orchards seemed to go on forever, and all those rich colors against the African terrain and the blue sky were breathtaking.

The freshly picked oranges were collected in big containers and loaded onto trucks. A little hatch opened in each truck, and the oranges went spilling into a washing area where people with hoses sprayed them clean. Then the oranges were rolled onto a conveyor belt and carried up to the facility. The rinds were grated away, and the oil was produced.

The producers make juice with the rest of the fruit, of course! Several clear tubes showed the tasty juice flowing from the press to storage containers. The vibrant colors and scent filled the facility and seemed to invigorate everyone there. They all had big smiles and bright eyes, and were happy to answer our questions. The energy in the entire place was very uplifting, just like citrus oils!

As if getting to see citrus essential oil production wasn't enough excitement, Jess and Clive surprised us with another invitation. We weren't far from a few friends of theirs who distilled tea tree essential oil. Did Christina and I want to take a side trip to meet the tea tree distillers and see more essential oil production?

Of course we did! I was thrilled. I'd been using tea tree essential oil since my earliest days of working with aromatherapy in the mid-1980s, and yet I had never visited a tea tree distiller. I'd always wanted to, but this was one distiller trip that never seemed to quite find its way onto my travel schedule.

I was finally going to meet this tree for the first time.

The *Melaleuca alternifolia* distillers were a couple who worked a huge plantation out in a gorgeous, hilly, rural area of South Africa. The tea trees themselves looked a bit like small pine trees but with soft needles. They filled the air with a clear, fresh scent, and they went on and on as far as I could see.

The farmers cut the branches with a charming old tractor, going row by row, and then trucked the harvest down to the stills, which the distillers had built themselves.

We got to know one another over the hour it took for the tea tree to be distilled. Like the other distillers that Jess and Clive worked with, the tea tree distillers didn't focus much on marketing. They simply lived in close connection with the land and their tea trees, distilling their oil for people who needed it. As we talked, the medicinal aroma of the tea tree oil filled the air and made everything feel magical. It was as though I was finally getting to meet a friend I had corresponded with for over 20 years.

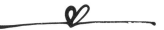

Thyme

Common name: Thyme
Latin name: *Thymus vulgaris* ct. linalool
Aroma: Fresh and herbal, with soft, woody undertones
Aromatic note: Top-Middle

THYME CT. LINALOOL'S GIFTS

You can think of thyme ct. linalool like a ballet dancer—graceful, sweet, beautiful, and very strong.

Thyme essential oil is excellent at bringing out your strength. It can support health, energy, and emotions, and it's able to do so in a particularly gentle way.

Research tells us that thyme has a powerful effect against infections and inflammation, and it's been used in this way for thousands of years. Soldiers in ancient Rome took invigorating thyme baths to feel brave and stay healthy, and thyme was used in hospital tents during WWI.

It's such a comforting oil to use when you have a cold or flu, or when you're suffering from allergies. It can soothe respiratory discomfort and help your body get rid of clogging mucus, while supporting you back to health. Thyme works well in diffusers, inhalers, and steam blends. In an inhaler with conifer essential oils, such as hemlock and black spruce, thyme can offer relief for sore throats since it can help reduce coughs and ease pain.

Some thyme chemotypes (for example, thyme ct. thymol) that are good for helping prevent and reduce infections can be harsh on skin, so it's important to blend them with skin-nourishing essential oils. However, skin irritation isn't such a concern with the linalool chemotype of thyme. Thyme ct. linalool is very skin-nourishing and a soothing choice for topical blends that help relieve pain, calm inflammation, and reduce infection. It adds softness and tenderness to blends that might otherwise be a little irritating. Try it with juniper or saro.

Emotionally, thyme ct. linalool helps you feel your inner strength. Its reassuring effects can restore your spirit and optimism if you're sick or are in pain.

Thyme essential oil is also useful in natural cleaning products.

You can use thyme for:

- Respiratory support
- Soothing allergies and clearing sinus congestion
- Easing sore throats and coughs
- Helping to clear infections
- Reducing swelling
- Soothing sore muscles and joints
- Energy, focus, and optimism

SPEND TIME WITH THYME WHEN YOU'RE SICK

Thyme loves being with people when they're not well and are in need of courage and support.

It visits patients in hospitals and clinics, spending time connecting with them so they feel happy, strong, and inspired. Sometimes Thyme has small gatherings in hospital community rooms, and other times it visits people one on one to cheer them up.

Thyme always seems to know exactly what a patient needs in order to feel strong. That's because it's a good listener. Thyme can tell if someone feels afraid (even if they don't want to admit it), and it reminds them of times when they were brave so they get in touch with their own strength. It can also tell if someone feels sad, and it shares inspiring stories while diffusing "feel better" aromatherapy blends. If a patient's body is sore and they feel like they'll never get well, Thyme offers a massage and reminds them of their body's innate ability to heal in amazing ways. If someone needs connection with friends, Thyme invites them to a small gathering or motivational workshop.

After "spending time with Thyme," people feel supported by life and confident in their ability to heal. They learn to see their fears as invitations to grow and to listen to their hearts when they feel uncertain. Nothing makes Thyme feel stronger than helping others to feel stronger too!

THYME'S SAFETY TIPS

Thyme's safety considerations depend on the chemotype (ct.). The linalool chemotype will not irritate skin and can be used safely. Read more about chemotypes on **page 109**.

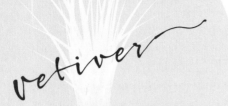

Common name: Vetiver

Latin name: *Vetiveria zizanoides*

Aroma: Deep, rich, and earthy. Strong, with hints of sweetness and wood. Can be quite smoky depending on the country of origin.

Aromatic note: Base

VETIVER'S STRENGTHS

Vetiver essential oil is so soothing that it's called "Oil of Tranquility" in some parts of the world. It's known to calm the nervous system and, therefore, support overall health.

Vetiver grass, vetiver hydrosol, and vetiver essential oil are all used for their relaxing aromas but in different ways.

On Réunion Island, the grass is woven into mats and window blinds, which smell sweetly fragrant in the rain and keep rooms cool naturally when breezes blow through.

The hydrosol can also be used to cool you down. Try it as a body mist, and be sure to get a few spritzes on the back of your neck.

Vetiver essential oil is enchanting all by itself (add a few drops to 1 oz (30 ml) of jojoba for a quick, simple perfume oil), and it blends well with many other aromas. Florals blend beautifully with vetiver, as do other base notes like patchouli. I especially like vetiver with rose and bergamot mint.

Many essential oils that are good for relaxation are also deeply nourishing to skin. Vetiver's soothing qualities help to calm skin irritation and inflammation, even for more chronic conditions that cause irritation. The essential oil is very thick and doesn't diffuse easily. It's perfect in a bath salt or body oil to use before bed. You can also try a linen spray with vetiver hydrosol.

You can use vetiver for:

- Daily skin care
- Rejuvenating damaged skin
- Soothing skin irritation
- Cooling
- Natural perfumes, particularly as an earthy base note
- Meditation and contemplation
- Feeling relaxed and uplifted

VETIVER'S NATURAL SLEEP CLINIC

If you have an "on again, off again" relationship with rest and relaxation, Vetiver warmly invites you to its natural sleep clinic.

People who come to Vetiver's clinic usually stay for a minivacation so Vetiver has time to help them get in touch with their body's natural rhythms of energy and relaxation. It knows rest isn't "one size fits all" and that different people need different things. That's why it has a variety of techniques available. Vetiver offers relaxation massages with body oils it makes itself, warm baths, the softest bed linens that smell so good and feel so comforting, and inhalers that you can keep with you to stay relaxed all day. It even leads group meditation sessions!

Vetiver doesn't just want to provide a "fix it and forget it" solution to sleep. It wants to help you get at the root of what isn't allowing you to really rest. It will sit down and chat with you, glad to help you talk through your troubles and find the topics that make you feel happy.

Sometimes these are things you may have lost touch with a long time ago. Vetiver, a root oil, is good at helping you "dig to the roots" of your heart!

VETIVER'S SAFETY TIPS

Vetiver is usually a very skin-safe essential oil, and is not generally known to cause irritation.

Common name: Ylang Ylang
Latin name: *Cananga odorata*
Aroma: Exotic, rich, heavy, sweet, and floral, with warm hints of spice
Aromatic note: Middle-Base

YLANG YLANG'S PASSION

Ylang ylang's aroma is intense, and a single drop goes a long way. It's often used for perfumes.

Ylang ylang has a reputation for creating harmony throughout the mind, heart, and body. Research shows it's excellent for helping the nervous system relax. A particular effect of ylang ylang is calming a rapid heartbeat. It can also help your mind relax so you can rest more easily. This is a great essential oil for meditation blends with frankincense or patchouli, and for blends to help you unwind when it's time for bed.

Physical tension responds to ylang ylang in the same way as emotional tension—it simply melts away. An inhaler with ylang ylang essential oil can help you relax so deeply that your muscles release any feelings of tightness they've been holding. This applies to digestion blends too. In blends for digestion and stomach cramps, ylang ylang pairs well with lime, bergamot mint, and ginger.

In places such as Madagascar and Java, where ylang ylang trees grow naturally, there is a tradition of using it for skin and hair care. Try ylang ylang in a bath salt before bed, or in a body oil, hand soap, or salve for moisturizing dry skin.

Ylang ylang can help with:

- Calming your heart and encouraging trust
- Daily skin care
- Soothing skin irritation
- Calming inflammation
- Soothing sore muscles
- Supporting digestion
- Natural perfume blends
- Meditation and contemplation

YLANG YLANG'S "EXOTIC HYPNOTIC" MADAGASCAR MUSIC STUDIO

Ylang Ylang has a talent for expressing itself. It grows aromatic flowers that can fill a whole yard with gorgeous scent and make everyone feel peaceful. It also loves playing music that can have the same effect.

Ylang Ylang's friends say its music is so relaxing, it's almost hypnotic. They encouraged it to open its own recording studio. Have you ever listened to a piece of music that dissolved your stress like magic and seemed to transport you to a place of complete peace? Maybe it even lulled you to sleep?

That song might have come out of Ylang Ylang's recording studio in Madagascar!

Ylang Ylang's friends from all over the world come to collaborate on songs. The studio's beautiful location inspires creativity, and Ylang Ylang burns handmade incense during recording sessions to help everyone get in a relaxed, creative state of mind. After a great jam session, everyone shares a big meal full of easy-to-digest foods and relaxes in Ylang Ylang's outdoor hot tub. It makes its own skin-nourishing body products for friends to use after they dry off their skin.

The soothing, nourishing atmosphere where Ylang Ylang and its friends create art together infuses into the music on its albums, and its fans appreciate that . . . until they fall asleep!

YLANG YLANG'S SAFETY TIPS

Ylang ylang may be skin-sensitizing. In their book *Essential Oil Safety*, Robert Tisserand and Rodney Young suggest staying at a maximum dilution of 0.8% when blending with ylang ylang for topical use, and they caution against using it on hypersensitive, diseased, or damaged skin.

Using more than a few drops of ylang ylang can sometimes cause nausea or headaches. To sidestep this, use only one or two drops in your blends.

Ylang ylang is known to very slightly lower blood pressure. To be extra cautious, you may want to choose a different essential oil if you're blending for someone who already has low blood pressure. You can use lavender instead.

Common name: Yuzu
Latin name: *Citrus junos*
Aroma: Citrusy and radiant, with hints of grapefruit, bergamot, and mandarin
Aromatic note: Top

YUZU'S FLAIR

Yuzu is a Japanese citrus fruit that looks like a small orange with a bumpy rind. In Japan, it's considered a fruit of new beginnings and vibrant health, and taking a hot bath with yuzu is a tradition on the winter solstice. The goal is to release the aroma of the fruit and infuse the water with yuzu's therapeutic properties. Sometimes the whole fruits are dropped right into the water! An aromatic yuzu bath can warm the body, calm the mind, and leave you feeling inspired for the future.

The essential oil can have the same effects. Yuzu is a comforting addition to blends meant to soothe anxiety. Its emotional qualities are similar to those of sweet orange, so while yuzu is uplifting, it's also right for bedtime blends.

Yuzu baths are also said to protect against colds and to help reduce infections. It's very soothing to the respiratory system, and can help your body calm inflammation and break up congestion. I've also used yuzu in blends for body aches that can accompany winter colds or the flu.

Like the other citrus essential oils, yuzu is helpful for stomach issues. Try it in a bath salt or belly oil for digestion. Its ability to calm inflammation and ease muscle spasms can offer a sense of relief.

You can use yuzu for:

- Respiratory support
- Clearing mucus and congestion
- Helping to clear infections
- Calming inflammation
- Supporting digestion
- Easing nausea
- Soothing sore muscles
- Feeling relaxed and uplifted

YUZU'S NEW YEAR'S BLAST PARTIES

Every year on the winter solstice, Yuzu throws the biggest New Year's party in town!

People come dressed up as something they want to be or do in the coming year. Are you going to go snorkeling with dolphins? Come wearing a scuba mask and flippers! Maybe you're planning on starting a career as an aromatherapist. Come to the party wearing perfume you've made yourself!

Yuzu has big banquet tables full of foods from all over the world. Feel free to kick off your new year by trying new things—the ends of every banquet table are stocked with baskets of homemade digestion blends. It also has a few swimming pools outside, and those are some of the most popular party areas. You can splash with friends in the "cool pool," then relax in the "hot springs" with whole citrus fruits floating in the water around you.

After the turn of the year, Yuzu turns the energetic music to more soothing songs, and diffuses uplifting essential oil blends that help everyone calm down and rest.

Yuzu loves winter parties, but its doors are open all year for any friends who need to take a little time for themselves, refresh their outlook on life, and rejuvenate their health.

YUZU'S SAFETY TIPS

Yuzu essential oil is not phototoxic. Citrus trees can be heavily sprayed with pesticides, which come through the cold-pressing process and are found in the essential oil. I recommend buying yuzu oil produced from organically grown fruit.

Recipes

Now that you've met 40 different essential oils, you can get to know them better by actively blending with them for different purposes.

You'll find that some of these recipes have similar uses. For example, there are several hand cleanser blends that reduce germs. In places where you see multiple blends for similar purposes, you can choose whichever blend looks most appealing to you or includes oils that you already know you like. Sometimes one blend will work wonders for you, while the other may not get the results you want. This is normal, and it varies from person to person.

Some of these recipes can be used on a daily basis, and others you may want to keep around in case of unexpected situations like sunburns, rashes, or respiratory infections.

You'll also find recipes here made with hydrosols (aromatic waters that have therapeutic effects) and natural carrier oils, butters, and waxes. They are all deeply supportive of skin's health even without essential oils blended into them. Recipes made with just hydrosols or carriers can be perfect for people who have sensitivity issues—such as people who don't like strong aromas or with delicate or compromised immune systems. They're also gentle enough for very small children.

Many of the essential oil skin-care recipes will direct you back to the same foundational body butter or firm salve blend to use as the base. While the base of these recipes is the same, the various essential oil blends create different effects. The foundational "Luxurious Body Butter" recipe is on **page 135**, and the "Firm Salve" recipe is on **page 136**. These two foundational recipes will serve you well in your blending.

You can also get creative with blending the carriers themselves to create different body butters and firm salves. Once you get comfortable blending, there is no end to the kinds of products you can make and the essential oil combinations you can add. It's a foundation of knowledge that gives you a lot of room for personalizing your blends and creating products that support your unique needs and preferences.

Every recipe in the book includes an adjusted version for children with kid-friendly essential oil substitutions and dilutions.

Before you make any of the recipes, be sure to check both the shelf lives of your ingredients so you know how long your product will last and any safety concerns for the essential oils.

HYDROSOLS

Watching the process of distillation is fascinating, because you can see the hydrosol and essential oil both collecting in the same vessel. The hydrosol fills most of the collection vessel, and the essential oil is a thin layer, usually floating right on top of the hydrosol since oil and water don't mix.

Like essential oils, hydrosols have a variety of therapeutic effects. They can be energizing, relaxing, soothing to burns, or calming to inflammation. Some hydrosols can even help to reduce infections. German chamomile and lavender hydrosols are so gentle, safe, and effective that I like to use them for small children and babies. Hydrosols don't come with the same safety concerns associated with essential oils.

The hydrosol and essential oil from the same plant often have similar properties, but they can also have some different properties, simply because the components in the oil are different from those in the hydrosol. The essential oil and hydrosol often smell different too.

You can use hydrosols for cleaning products, facial washes, skin care, clay masks, after-sun sprays, and more. You'll find a lot of recipes throughout this book using the following hydrosols:

- **Frankincense** – Frankincense hydrosol is deeply nourishing for skin that's irritated or inflamed. Its earthy, grounding aroma helps inspire calm and is wonderful in a bedtime body spray or linen spray.

- **German Chamomile** – German chamomile hydrosol is also deeply nourishing for skin that's irritated or inflamed. Most people with sensitive skin find German chamomile hydrosol soothing and healing. It's popular for children and babies, and a few spritzes in a bathtub (for adults or kids) can be very relaxing.

- **Lavender** – Lavender hydrosol smells amazing, with a calming, reassuring floral aroma. It's a very versatile hydrosol—skin loves it. It's wonderful for emotional support and effective in natural cleaning blends, including some carpet and upholstery sprays that can really freshen up a room.

- **Neroli** – Neroli hydrosol has a beautiful aroma and is very loving to skin. It's calming and comforting, and works well as a perfume and skin-care mist.

- **Peppermint** – Peppermint hydrosol is nice and cooling. A few spritzes on the back of your neck can help you cool down on a hot day. It's also a strong ingredient in blends for itchy skin and is an effective cleaner, air freshener, and insect repellent.

- **Rose** – Rose hydrosol is probably most famous for its role in facial care. It smells rich and floral and when spritzed on your skin, it hydrates, soothes irritation, calms redness, and nurtures skin's overall appearance.

- **Tea Tree** – Tea tree hydrosol is excellent in blends for natural cleaning and is nice to your skin. It helps keep cuts and scrapes clean too.

- **Vetiver** – Vetiver hydrosol has a strong earthy aroma and a relaxing presence. It's slightly cooling on skin, and can calm irritation and support skin's overall health.

AROMATHERAPY INHALERS

There are two methods to make the aromatherapy inhaler recipes in this book.

The first is to put the cotton insert into the inhaler's sleeve and drop your essential oils right onto the cotton. This method is convenient if you know the exact essential oil blend.

The second method is helpful if you're creating a blend drop by drop. In this case, drop the essential oils into a little bowl before soaking the cotton insert in them. This way you can adjust the aroma of the blend as you create it. I suggest using about 15 drops of essential oil total in an inhaler. There will be a small amount of essential oil left over in the little bowl. Instead of washing it out right away, you can leave it out on your counter to let the essential oils evaporate into the air. They'll make the room smell amazing!

STOVETOP MELTING METHOD

You'll find a lot of recipes for body butters and salves in this book. To make them, you'll need to melt natural butters and oils with beeswax. Depending on the texture of your ingredients and how much beeswax you add, you can create a variety of consistencies.

Once you know how to make a foundational body butter recipe, you can add essential oils to achieve different effects. You can make body butters to help you relax, soothe skin irritation, help yourself heal, reduce infections (including in your respiratory system), inspire focus and concentration, ease digestion, and more. No matter what you're using your body butter for, you'll know that the body butter itself will be skin-nourishing!

I'm going to share two foundational body butters that will work well for all of the recipes in this book. One is softer, so you can make rich, luxurious body butters. The other is firmer, perfect for salves and balms. Each of these recipes will give you more than one jar of body butter and salve. I find this very convenient so you don't have to make a new batch every time you want to make a blend. You don't have to add essential oils immediately to every jar, and you can always remelt a jar of body butter and add essential oils at a later date.

To remelt a glass jar of body butter or salve, all you have to do is put a small pot of water on the stove and bring it to a simmer, and then carefully set your jar, with the lid still on, in the water. You won't need much water—it should reach only about halfway up your glass jar and shouldn't touch the rim.

When the butter or salve is melted, you can remove the jar from the heat, stir in the essential oils, and let the blend resolidify. This process can be done only with body butters in glass jars, as the heat would melt a PET plastic jar.

Most of the recipes in this book for body butters, salves, and balms will refer you back to one of these two foundational blends. You can bookmark this page, or copy it and keep a printed version in your kitchen for easy reference. You don't need any special equipment. You can make both of these recipes right in your kitchen on your stove, using utensils you probably already have. That's why I call this the "Stovetop Melting Method." All you need is:

- A wide cooking pot (3 quarts (2.8 liters) should be plenty of room.)
- A 16 oz (480 ml) Pyrex measuring cup with a handle (Your Pyrex has to fit inside your pot.)
- A glass stirring rod or the handle of a stainless-steel spoon
- Your stove

STOVETOP MELTING METHOD SETUP

- Fill the cooking pot about one-fourth of the way with water and bring it to a low, simmering boil.

- Place the Pyrex measuring cup in the pot so the water heats the outside of it and the handle is hanging over the edge of the pot. Leaving the handle outside of the pot will prevent it from getting so hot that it burns your hand.

- The water shouldn't be boiling so strongly that it splatters into the Pyrex cup. You're going to melt your ingredients in the Pyrex, and you want to keep water out of it. This setup acts as a makeshift double boiler.

- Weigh or measure all your ingredients so they're ready to put in the Pyrex. You can use a graduated cylinder or kitchen scale. The "tare" function on a kitchen scale allows you to weigh your bowl first and reset the weight to "0" before you put your ingredients in the bowl.

When you're not standing at your stove, you can work on any surface you like. Your work space can be your kitchen counter next to your sink, your dining room table, or a craft room. If you want to protect your work surface, you can use a silicone mat found at any kitchen supply store.

Here are the body butter and salve recipes that form the base for many recipes in this book. You can find the ingredients in Aromatherapy Resources on **page 255**.

Luxurious Body Butter

This recipe makes 7 oz (196 g) of body butter. You'll need four 2 oz (60 ml) glass jars.

INGREDIENTS

1 oz (28 g) beeswax (*Cera alba*)

2 oz (60 ml) jojoba (*Simmondsia chinensis*)

2 oz (56 g) cocoa butter (*Theobroma cacao*)

2 oz (56 g) coconut oil (*Cocos nucifera*)

DIRECTIONS

Follow the Stovetop Melting Method Setup directions on **pages 133–134**.

Add the beeswax to your Pyrex first. It will take the longest to melt since it's the hardest ingredient.

Once your beeswax is melted, add the jojoba. Your melted waxes may resolidify a bit, but they'll melt again quickly. You can stir your blend gently with your glass stirring rod or the handle of your spoon.

Add the cocoa butter and melt.

Add the coconut oil and melt.

Be sure to stay by the stove until the blend is melted.

As soon as all the ingredients are melted together, remove the blend from the heat. If you're adding essential oils, now is the time to stir them in.

Pour the blend into the glass jars and cover them. It won't take long (about 15 minutes) for it to solidify.

Firm Salve

This recipe makes 5 oz (140 g) of a slightly firmer balm. You can use three 2 oz (60 ml) jars.

INGREDIENTS

1 oz (28 g) beeswax (*Cera alba*)

1 oz (30 ml) jojoba (*Simmondsia chinensis*)

2 oz (56 g) cocoa butter (*Theobroma cacao*)

1 oz (28 g) coconut oil (*Cocos nucifera*)

DIRECTIONS

Follow the Stovetop Melting Method Setup on **pages 133–134**.

Melt the beeswax in the Pyrex measuring cup.

Add the jojoba and remelt. You can stir gently with your glass stirring rod or the handle of your spoon, if you like.

Add the cocoa butter.

Add the coconut oil.

Stir gently until all ingredients are melted.

Remove the blend from the heat. If you're adding essential oils, now is the time to stir them in.

Pour the blend into the glass jars and cover.

You'll notice that for both blends, the melting process starts with the beeswax, which is the hardest ingredient in the list. Then we add jojoba, which is also a wax and withstands heat well. After that, we add ingredients according to how firm they are. Cocoa butter comes next, followed by the coconut oil, which is the softest ingredient in the list. If we were working with another liquid, such as avocado oil, it would be added last. Basically, the more heat-sensitive the ingredient, the later in the process it gets added to the blend.

Always be careful when you're working with hot, liquefied butters and oils. Use the same caution you would use when cooking food. Keep your attention on your blend (no multitasking!), and you'll be fine.

Cleaning up is easy. If there's any excess butter or oil on your utensils and surfaces, wipe them down with a paper towel. Then use hot water and dishwashing liquid.

Have fun blending!

skin care

Your skin is the largest organ on your body, and a significant point of connection with the world.

Skin can be very sensitive. You can always rely on it to tell you when something "rubs it the wrong way." If your skin becomes uncomfortable, dry, or irritated, it can make everything that touches you feel uncomfortable. If your skin is not happy, it's not easy for the rest of you to be happy!

Using an all-natural, organic, unprocessed skin-care approach can keep your skin extremely happy. It's not always easy to find products like this. Even some of the purest products sold in health-food stores may have been sitting on the shelf for a while. Sometimes these products can create more negative reactions than positive ones.

That's why I'm such a fan of making my own skin-care products. I always know where my ingredients come from, what their shelf lives are, and how my skin is going to react to them.

Your blends can nourish and moisturize, reduce oiliness, and soothe ongoing conditions. Depending on the essential oils you use, your skin care can help you feel meditative and relaxed, or energized and ready to go. You can even make shower gels and face washes that don't require any soap. (Argan oil makes a luxurious face wash!)

Nobody knows your skin better than you. When you make your own skin-care products, you can work with the oils and ingredients that help your unique skin feel and look its best.

Geranium and Cedarwood's "Skin Silk" Soap-Free Face Wash

Geranium has sensitive skin that gets dried out and irritated from using soap. It created this light, silky, soap-free face wash to cleanse and moisturize its skin instead.

Use this recipe: to cleanse, moisturize, and nourish skin without soap.

2 oz (60 ml) argan oil

1 drop cedarwood

1 drop geranium

1 drop opopanax

DIRECTIONS

Make the blend in a 2 oz (60 ml) glass bottle. Pour the argan oil into the bottle, and add the essential oils.

FOR KIDS 💚

The version for kids is the same as the one for grown-ups.

Neroli and Frankincense's "Pretty Peaceful" Soap-Free Face Wash

Peaceful Frankincense and enchanting Neroli have been making skin-care blends for hundreds of years. Their soap-free face wash cleanses, moisturizes, and calms irritation so skin feels pretty and peaceful.

Use this recipe: to cleanse, moisturize, nourish, and calm irritation to skin without soap.

1 oz (30 ml) argan oil

1 oz (28 g) aloe vera gel

1 drop neroli

1 drop frankincense

DIRECTIONS

Make the blend in a 2 oz (60 ml) glass bottle. Pour the argan oil and aloe vera into the bottle, and add the essential oils.

Shake the blend gently before each use.

FOR KIDS ♡

The version for kids is the same as the one for grown-ups.

Skin Care

DIRECTIONS FOR FACIAL MISTS

Simply blend the hydrosols in a 4 oz (120 ml) glass spray bottle.

I recommend making these blends fresh every few weeks.

Vetiver's
"Tranquil Rose"
Facial Mist

Vetiver made this facial mist for hydrating and healing sensitive skin. A few spritzes feel especially revitalizing on warm days.

Use this recipe: to hydrate your face, cool down redness, calm inflammation, and heal sensitive skin.

3½ oz (105 ml) vetiver hydrosol

½ oz (15 ml) rose hydrosol

Neroli and Frankincense's
"Pretty Peaceful" Facial Mist

Frankincense and Neroli made this hydrating facial mist to follow up their "Pretty Peaceful" Soap-Free Face Wash. Spritz it on after washing your face and anytime throughout the day.

Use this recipe: to hydrate, cool, and nourish skin.

3 oz (90 ml) neroli hydrosol

1 oz (30 ml) frankincense hydrosol

FOR KIDS ♡

The versions for kids are the same as the ones for grown-ups.

ROSE'S
"WHITE BLOSSOM"
EXFOLIATING FACE CLEANSER

This is Rose's love poem to your skin. The white clay offers a gentle scrub, the avocado oil cleanses and moisturizes, and Rose itself nourishes and heals.

Use this recipe: to gently exfoliate, cleanse, and nourish your face.

1 oz (28 g) white clay

1 oz (30 ml) avocado oil

1 drop rose

DIRECTIONS

Use a 2 oz (60 ml) glass jar for this blend. Blend the white clay and avocado oil in the jar, stirring with a glass stirring rod or the handle of a stainless-steel spoon. Then add the drop of rose oil and stir again.

FOR KIDS 💚

The version for kids is the same as the one for grown-ups.

Myrrh's "Blessings and Beauty" Skin Spa Butter

Myrrh's "Blessings and Beauty" body butter is like a spa treatment for skin. Use it daily for skin that feels parched, itchy, and in need of extra nourishment.

Use this recipe: to protect and heal chronically dry, itchy, and irritated skin.

7 oz (196 g) Luxurious Body Butter (**page 135**)

38 drops myrrh

18 drops geranium

28 drops helichrysum

DIRECTIONS

Use four 2 oz (60 ml) glass jars when making the Luxurious Body Butter on **page 135**. If you have a graduated cylinder, you can measure out the essential oils while the body butter is melting over the stove. If not, blend them drop by drop in a small bowl. Then pour the essential oil blend into the melted body butter, and carefully pour the mixture into the glass jars.

FOR KIDS ♡

Substitute:

7 oz (196 g) Luxurious Body Butter (**page 135**)

19 drops myrrh

9 drops geranium

14 drops helichrysum

PALMAROSA'S "SUPER SOAKER" DRY SPOT SALVE

Palmarosa's hands were dry, cracked, and painful. Its usual moisturizer wasn't quite healing enough, so it created this "Super Soaker" salve to save the day.

Use this recipe: to moisturize spots of dry, cracked skin.

5 oz (140 g) Firm Salve (**page 136**)

19 drops palmarosa

15 drops myrrh

13 drops ylang ylang

DIRECTIONS

Use three 2 oz (60 ml) glass jars when making the Firm Salve on **page 136**. If you have a graduated cylinder, you can measure out the essential oils while the salve is melting over the stove. If not, blend them drop by drop in a small bowl. Then pour the essential oil blend into the melted body butter, and carefully pour the melted mixture into the glass jars.

FOR KIDS 💜

5 oz (140 g) Firm Salve (**page 136**)

12 drops palmarosa

9 drops myrrh

8 drops ylang ylang

Skin Care

Cedarwood's "Roots and Wood" Bath Salt

Cedarwood had an exciting day and made this bath salt to help it calm down in the evening. This blend is perfect for right before bed.

Use this recipe: to relax and nurture your spirit at the end of the day.

2 oz (56 g) salt

1 teaspoon (5 ml) jojoba

3 drops cedarwood

2 drops vetiver

DIRECTIONS

Use a 2 oz (60 ml) glass jar for this blend.

Put the salt into the jar. Blend the jojoba and essential oils in a separate bowl before adding to the salt. Stir with a glass stirring rod or the handle of a stainless-steel spoon.

This recipe makes enough for one bath. If you love it, you can make more and store it in a glass jar. The jojoba provides a skin-nourishing carrier to distribute the essential oils.

I recommend making this blend fresh every few weeks.

Pay attention to your skin's responses when using essential oils in a bath. What's comfortable for you may be different from what's comfortable for other people. You may want more jojoba, less essential oil, or even different essential oils from the ones in the recipe.

I suggest using about five drops of essential oil total in a bath.

FOR KIDS

Substitute:

2 oz (56 g) salt

1 teaspoon (5 ml) jojoba

2 drops cedarwood

1 drop vetiver

Frankincense and Myrrh's
"The Perfect Marriage" Shower Gel

Frankincense and Myrrh are the perfect pair—they're both distilled from resins and love to care for skin, deepen the breath, and center the mind. Nobody was surprised when they decided to get married!

Use this recipe: to cleanse and heal your skin and calm your mind in the shower.

1 oz (28 g) aloe vera gel

8 drops myrrh

5 drops frankincense

DIRECTIONS

Make the blend in a 1 oz (30 ml) flip-top bottle. Pour the aloe vera into the bottle and add the essential oils.

Shake gently before each use to help distribute the essential oils through the aloe.

I recommend making this blend fresh every few weeks.

FOR KIDS 💙

Substitute:

1 oz (28 g) aloe vera gel

4 drops myrrh

2 drops frankincense

Skin Care

Avocado's
"Sweet Brown and Deep Green"
Sugar Scrub

. . . .

Avocado oil has a talent for absorbing deeply into skin and restoring it through and through. It created this blend to offer that level of protection as it cleanses and scrubs skin smooth.

. . . .

Use this recipe: to gently exfoliate and cleanse your skin while restoring it.

3 oz (84 g) brown sugar

1 oz (30 ml) avocado oil

10 drops vetiver

10 drops patchouli

10 drops Roman chamomile

DIRECTIONS

Use a 4 oz (120 ml) PET plastic jar for this blend.

Put the brown sugar into the jar. Blend the avocado oil and essential oils in a separate bowl. Pour the oil mixture into the brown sugar, and stir with a glass stirring rod or the handle of a stainless-steel spoon.

Use a small handful in your bath or shower.

I recommend making this blend fresh every few weeks.

FOR KIDS 💚

Substitute:

3 oz (84 g) brown sugar   5 drops patchouli

1 oz (30 ml) avocado oil   5 drops Roman chamomile

5 drops vetiver

Castile's "Essentially Clean" Foam Hand Soaps

Castile soap wanted a natural foam soap for every occasion. These recipes are right for bathrooms, kitchens, travel kits, yoga studios, and massage offices.

Use this recipe: to clean your hands, reduce infections, and support skin.

Frankincense's "Deserts and Forests" Foam Soap

1.4 oz (40 ml) castile soap

7 drops geranium

7 drops frankincense

6 drops cedarwood

4 drops opopanax

Rosalina's "Lavender, Lavender Tea Tree, and Tea Tree" Foam Soap

1.4 oz (40 ml) castile soap

8 drops lavender

8 drops tea tree

8 drops rosalina

Palmarosa's "Ylang-arosa Bouquet" Foam Soap

1.4 oz (40 ml) castile soap

8 drops ylang ylang

8 drops palmarosa

DIRECTIONS

Use a 50 ml foam soap pump bottle. There will be extra space in the top of the bottle to allow room for the pump itself.

FOR KIDS

Use the same amount of castile soap but reduce the amount of essential oils by about half, as below.

FRANKINCENSE'S "DESERTS AND FORESTS" FOAM SOAP

1.4 oz (40 ml) castile soap

3 drops geranium

4 drops frankincense

3 drops cedarwood

2 drops opopanax

ROSALINA'S "LAVENDER, LAVENDER TEA TREE, AND TEA TREE" FOAM SOAP

1.4 oz (40 ml) castile soap

4 drops lavender

4 drops tea tree

4 drops rosalina

PALMAROSA'S "YLANG-AROSA BOUQUET" FOAM SOAP

1.4 (40 ml) castile soap

4 drops ylang ylang

4 drops palmarosa

ALOE VERA'S "KISS AWAY THE SUN" SPRAY

Aloe Vera loves restoring skin that's seen too much sun. It keeps this blend in the refrigerator to create a cooling sensation.

Use this recipe: to cool and soothe skin, especially sunburned skin.

1 oz (28 g) aloe vera gel

4 drops lavender

4 drops helichrysum

4 drops German chamomile

DIRECTIONS

Make this blend in a 1 oz (30 ml) glass spray bottle. Pour the aloe vera into the bottle and add the essential oils.

Shake the blend gently before each use to help distribute the essential oils through the aloe.

I recommend making this blend fresh every few weeks.

FOR KIDS 🖤

Substitute:

1 oz (28 g) aloe vera gel

2 drops lavender

2 drops helichrysum

2 drops German chamomile

Skin Care

Cedarwood's "Bugs Don't Bug Me!" Lotion

Cedarwood has always been skilled at keeping bugs out of closets and drawers. With this lotion, it's finally found a way to repel them from skin too!

Use this recipe: to repel bugs and take care of skin.

2 oz (56 g) unscented lotion

14 drops cedarwood

11 drops patchouli

7 drops palo santo

4 drops kunzea

DIRECTIONS

Make this blend in a 2 oz (60 ml) glass jar. Put the lotion into the jar and stir in the essential oils.

I recommend making this blend fresh every few weeks.

FOR KIDS

Substitute:

2 oz (56 g) unscented lotion

7 drops cedarwood

3 drops patchouli

2 drops palo santo

Lavender's "Bugs Bugged Me a Little" Bite and Sting Blend

Lavender is dedicated to skin care. When a bug bites or stings and inflammation flares up, Lavender doubles up its attention to calm the itch and soothe the pain.

Use this recipe: to soothe swelling, pain, and itching from bug bites and stings.

1 oz (28 g) aloe vera gel

3 drops German chamomile

8 drops lavender

2 drops peppermint

5 drops helichrysum

DIRECTIONS

Make this blend in a 1 oz (30 ml) PET plastic flip-top bottle. Pour the aloe vera into the bottle and add the essential oils.

Shake the blend gently before each use to help distribute the essential oils through the aloe.

I recommend making this blend fresh every few weeks.

FOR KIDS

Substitute:

1 oz (28 g) aloe vera gel

1 drop German chamomile

3 drops lavender

2 drops helichrysum

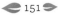

Skin Care

BEESWAX'S "BEE SWEET" LIP BALM

Beeswax has created a lip balm that tastes so sweet and feels so nourishing, it didn't need to add essential oils! The combination of beeswax, vanilla, and coconut oil are perfect.

Use this recipe: to keep your lips feeling smooth and moisturized.

1 oz (28 g) beeswax

1½ oz (45 ml) vanilla-infused jojoba

1½ oz (42 g) coconut oil

DIRECTIONS

Make your blend in four 1 oz (30 ml) lip balm tins or jars.

Set up the Stovetop Melting Method (**pages 133–134**).

Melt the beeswax in the Pyrex measuring cup.

Add the vanilla-infused jojoba.

Add the coconut oil and melt.

Pour the melted blend into tins or jars, and let them cool. It won't take long (about 15 minutes).

FOR KIDS

The version for kids is the same as the one for grown-ups.

Frankincense's "Nourished from Within" Body Oil

Frankincense has always been good at helping people feel cared for, protected, and supported from within. Its body oil offers those benefits to skin too.

Use this recipe: to moisturize, protect, and heal skin.

1 oz (30 ml) vanilla-infused jojoba

6 drops frankincense

4 drops myrrh

3 drops palo santo

2 drops rose

DIRECTIONS

Make the blend in a 1 oz (30 ml) glass bottle. Pour the jojoba into the bottle, and add the essential oils.

FOR KIDS 💜

Substitute:

1 oz (30 ml) vanilla-infused jojoba

2 drops frankincense

2 drops myrrh

1 drop palo santo

1 drop rose

Palmarosa's "Peaceful Earth" Body Oil

Along with nourishing skin, Palmarosa is also talented at helping people feel peaceful and grounded. It made this body oil to combine its many skills.

Use this recipe: to moisturize, protect, and heal skin.

1 oz (30 ml) jojoba

4 drops palmarosa

3 drops vetiver

3 drops patchouli

3 drops German chamomile

DIRECTIONS

Make the blend in a 1 oz (30 ml) glass bottle. Pour the jojoba into the bottle and add the essential oils.

FOR KIDS

Substitute:

1 oz (30 ml) jojoba

2 drops palmarosa

1 drop vetiver

1 drop patchouli

2 drops German chamomile

ALOE VERA AND COCONUT'S "DOUBLE-SWEET" DEODORANT

Aloe Vera and Coconut love when life smells sweet—naturally! They made a deodorant that's nourishing for sensitive skin and customizable with different essential oil blends.

Use this recipe: for an all-natural deodorant that's sweet to your body and your nose.

½ oz (14 g) coconut oil

½ oz (14 g) aloe vera gel

2 tablespoons (30 g) arrowroot powder

18 drops of essential oil (blend suggestions below)

DIRECTIONS

Make this blend in a 2 oz (60 ml) glass jar. Put the coconut oil and aloe vera together into the jar, and stir or mush them together gently with a small spoon. Then add the arrowroot powder and mush it gently into the blend.

Next, choose an essential oil blend from the next page to add. When you've chosen your oils, mush the drops gently into the deodorant.

Take a round cotton face pad, dab it into the deodorant, and apply it under your arms. You'll have to reapply it several times throughout the day because the ingredients are all-natural.

I recommend making this blend fresh every few weeks.

Patchouli's "Earthy Perfume" Blend

5 drops spike lavender

9 drops patchouli

4 drops neroli

Opopanax's "Resins Love Flowers" Blend

7 drops lavender

8 drops opopanax

3 drops rose

Neroli's "I Have Always Loved the Forest" Blend

10 drops neroli

4 drops piñon pine

4 drops juniper

FOR KIDS

These are great for kids' sweaty feet!

Substitute:

Patchouli's "Earthy Perfume" Blend

2 drops lavender

3 drop patchouli

1 drop neroli

Opopanax's "Resins Love Flowers" Blend

4 drops lavender

1 drops opopanax

1 drop rose

Neroli's "I Have Always Loved the Forest" Blend

3 drops neroli

1 drop piñon pine

1 drop juniper

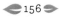

THE HYDROSOL TEAM'S "BATH BOOST"

The Hydrosols have a simple, fun way to make a bath feel more luxurious!

Use this recipe: to add skin-loving, aromatic hydrosol to your bath. Try:

- Rose hydrosol
- Vetiver hydrosol
- Frankincense hydrosol
- German chamomile hydrosol

Add a capful of hydrosol to your full bathtub, and then take your bath as usual . . . or maybe with a little more pleasure!

If you make a blend of hydrosols, I recommend making it fresh every few weeks.

FOR KIDS

The version for kids is the same as the one for grown-ups.

LAVENDER'S "HAPPIEST BABY EVER" SKIN-SOOTHING SPRAY

Lavender doesn't like to see babies and little kids suffer from baby acne and other skin irritation. It made this gentle and effective hydrosol spray to care for their skin.

Use this recipe: to soothe irritation, redness, and acne on a baby's skin or for children under five. Can be used as a diaper spray.

1 oz (30 ml) lavender hydrosol

1 oz (30 ml) German chamomile hydrosol

DIRECTIONS

Blend the hydrosols in a 2 oz (60 ml) glass spray bottle.

I recommend making this blend fresh every few weeks.

Argan's "Comforting Cocoa" Diaper Rash Butter

Argan oil loves taking care of little ones! It's very good at nourishing their sensitive skin without using any potentially harsh ingredients.

Use this recipe: to soothe painful diaper rash, and heal and protect a baby's skin.

¼ oz (7 g) beeswax

1 oz (30 ml) argan oil

½ oz (14 g) cocoa butter

DIRECTIONS

Make this blend in a 2 oz (60 ml) glass jar.

Set up the Stovetop Melting Method (**pages 133–134**).

Melt the beeswax in the Pyrex measuring cup.

Add the cocoa butter and melt.

When the beeswax and cocoa butter are melted together, add the argan oil and stir gently.

Remove the blend from the heat, pour it into the jar, and wait for it to cool (about 15 minutes).

Rest and Relaxation

Healthy sleep patterns play a big role in well-being.

When you get enough rest, everything in life seems to flow more easily. You have more focus, you can use your mind to the best of its ability, and your emotions feel more balanced. You can face what the day brings from a place of peace and confidence. Sleep can help your physical body feel healthier too. You can experience this when you go to sleep with a slight headache and wake up to find it completely gone.

Essential oils are comforting friends when you need a little support getting enough rest. You can use essential oils to help you fall asleep and stay asleep. Using oils to stay calm and centered during a busy, stressful day can actually help you be more productive, and the calmer you feel throughout the day, the easier it will be to get to sleep.

This chapter includes plenty of recipes and ideas for how to use essential oils and hydrosols to support healthy sleep. You can make bath salt blends and use them in a warm evening bath. Linen sprays are nice because they can make you feel like you're folding yourself up in a big aromatic hug as you tuck yourself into bed. Body butters and massage oils can help reduce physical tension while the aromas soothe and comfort you. There's a lot of room to be creative!

A great way to use the oils at night, especially if you'd like to use them as you're falling asleep, is with a diffuser. A diffuser distributes the essentials oils throughout the air in your room. You'll be inhaling the essential oils, and the entire room will smell amazing. Diffusing certain oils allows you to create a very warm, welcoming atmosphere, while other oils help to clean the air. Some oils do both.

Before you make any of the following recipes, be sure to check the shelf lives of your ingredients so you know how long your product will last and any safety concerns for the essential oils.

Orange's "Sweet Retreat" Diffuser Blend

Orange made this diffuser blend so you can create your own "miniretreat" whenever you need to feel relaxed and uplifted.

Use this recipe: anytime you want to rest and relax.

4 drops gingergrass

4 drops orange

2 drops geranium

DIRECTIONS

Simply drop all the essential oils into the diffuser.

FOR KIDS

Substitute:

2 drops gingergrass

2 drops orange

1 drop geranium

Frankincense's
"Frankly Relaxing" Diffuser Blend

Frankincense meditated for a long time on what to name this diffuser blend. "Calm as Chamomile?" "Frankin-chamomile?" What name could possibly convey how frankly relaxing this blend is?

Use this recipe: to relax your body and center your mind.

4 drops cedarwood

1 drop Roman chamomile

5 drops frankincense

DIRECTIONS

Simply drop all the essential oils into the diffuser.

FOR KIDS ♥

Substitute:

2 drops cedarwood

1 drop Roman chamomile

2 drops frankincense

Vetiver's "Root of Relaxation" Body Oil

Vetiver uses this skin-loving body oil to give its friends relaxing massages. It's so effective that sometimes they fall asleep on the massage table!

Use this recipe: as a moisturizing body oil or massage oil that helps you relax.

1 oz (30 ml) jojoba

5 drops vetiver

4 drops neroli

3 drops lavender

DIRECTIONS

Make the blend in a 1 oz (30 ml) glass bottle. Pour the jojoba into the bottle, and add the essential oils. Massage yourself with it to wind down at the end of the day.

FOR KIDS

Substitute:

1 oz (30 ml) jojoba

2 drops vetiver

1 drop neroli

2 drops lavender

Opopanax's "Relax All Day" Inhaler

Opopanax stays busy, but that doesn't mean it becomes stressed. This inhaler makes everything it does feel like a meditation.

Use this recipe: to stay relaxed in the middle of a busy day.

6 drops opopanax

3 drops palmarosa

2 drops basil ct. linalool

4 drops yuzu

DIRECTIONS

Add all the essential oil drops to the cotton component of an aromatherapy inhaler.

FOR KIDS

Substitute:

1 drop palmarosa

1 drop basil ct. linalool

3 drops opopanax

2 drops yuzu

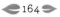

Lavender's "I'm Grateful for My Bed" Inhaler

Lavender sits down with this inhaler every night before bed, breathing deeply and thinking about all the things it's grateful for that happened that day.

Use this recipe: to prepare your heart and body for deep, restorative sleep.

2 drops ylang ylang

3 drops spikenard

4 drops vetiver

6 drops lavender

DIRECTIONS

Add all the essential oil drops to the cotton component of an aromatherapy inhaler.

FOR KIDS 💚

Substitute:

1 drop ylang ylang

1 drop spikenard

2 drops vetiver

3 drops lavender

Roman Chamomile's "I Need a Nap" Inhaler and Diffuser Blend

To get some quick, restorative rest in the middle of the day, Roman Chamomile combines a relaxing inhaler and diffuser blend.

Use this recipe: to restore yourself with a quick nap or a few moments of calm.

Inhaler

3 drops patchouli

5 drops orange

8 drops Roman chamomile

Diffuser Blend

2 drops ylang ylang

4 drops orange

3 drops Roman chamomile

DIRECTIONS

For the aromatherapy inhaler, add all the essential oil drops to the cotton component.

For the diffuser, simply drop all the essential oils into the diffuser.

FOR KIDS ♥

Substitute:

Inhaler

1 drop patchouli

2 drops orange

4 drops Roman chamomile

Diffuser Blend

1 drop ylang ylang

2 drops orange

2 drops Roman chamomile

Patchouli's "Peace Out" Bath Salt

For Patchouli, caring for its skin and restoring its spirit are one and the same. It made this bath salt to offer that experience to its friends too.

Use this recipe: to care for your skin and your sense of inner peace.

2 oz (56 g) salt

1 teaspoon (5 ml) vanilla-infused jojoba 2 drops cedarwood

2 drops patchouli

1 drop geranium

DIRECTIONS

Use a 2 oz (60 ml) glass jar for this blend.

Put the salt into the jar. Blend the jojoba and essential oils in a separate bowl before adding to the salt. Stir with a glass stirring rod or the handle of a stainless-steel spoon.

Use the whole thing in a bath and peace out!

This recipe makes enough for one bath. If you love it, you can make more and store it in a glass jar. The vanilla-infused jojoba provides a skin-nourishing carrier to distribute the essential oils.

Pay attention to your skin's responses when using essential oils in a bath. What's comfortable for you may be different from what's comfortable for other people. You may want more

jojoba, less essential oil, or different essential oils from the ones in the recipe.

I suggest using about five drops of essential oil total in a bath.

I recommend making this blend fresh every few weeks.

FOR KIDS

Substitute:

2 oz (56 g) salt

1 teaspoon (5 ml) vanilla-infused jojoba

1 drop cedarwood

1 drop patchouli

1 drop geranium

Neroli's "Seems Like a Dream" Linen Spray

Neroli loves to cuddle up and relax at bedtime, especially in sheets that are scented like flowers and resin. Talk about sweet dreams!

Use this recipe: for citrusy floral-scented sheets that are comforting at the end of the day.

2 oz (60 ml) neroli hydrosol

5 drops neroli

7 drops opopanax

DIRECTIONS

Use a 2 oz (60 ml) glass bottle for this blend. Combine all the ingredients in the bottle, give it a shake, and spritz your sheets and under your pillowcases with it.

I recommend making this blend fresh every few weeks.

FOR KIDS ♡

Substitute:

2 oz (60 ml) neroli hydrosol

2 drops neroli

3 drops opopanax

Vetiver's "Forever Vetiver" Linen Spray

One of Vetiver's most popular relaxation products is also its simplest—a pure hydrosol!

Use this recipe: for a rich and woody linen spray that helps you rest.

2 oz (60 ml) vetiver hydrosol

DIRECTIONS

Use a 2 oz (60 ml) glass bottle for this blend. Pour the vetiver hydrosol in the bottle and spritz your sheets and under your pillowcases with it.

Be sure to check with your supplier about the shelf life of your hydrosol.

FOR KIDS

The version for kids is the same as the one for grown-ups.

ROSE'S "ROLL-ON RADIANCE" PERFUME

Rose used to hand out rose-colored glasses to all its friends to help them see the world in a warm and loving light. Now it hands out roll-on bottles of this perfume, which work even better than the glasses.

Use this recipe: as a perfume that helps to inspire self-love and open your heart.

0.30 oz (about 9 ml) jojoba

1 drop rose

DIRECTIONS

Use a small 10 ml glass roll-on bottle. Pour the jojoba into the bottle, add a single drop of rose, snap the roller-top into place, and roll the blend onto your skin.

I recommend making this blend fresh every few weeks.

FOR KIDS

The version for kids is the same as the one for grown-ups.

CEDARWOOD'S "SOOTHE YOU THROUGH AND THROUGH" BODY BUTTER

Cedarwood made this body butter to soothe your whole being. It revitalizes skin, relaxes muscles, calms the mind, and inspires a happy heart.

Use this recipe: to nourish skin, ease tight muscles, and feel relaxed.

7 oz (196 g) Luxurious Body Butter (**page 135**)

11 drops neroli

15 drops patchouli

31 drops cedarwood

27 drops gingergrass

DIRECTIONS

Use four 2 oz (60 ml) glass jars when making the Luxurious Body Butter (**page 135**). If you have a graduated cylinder, you can measure out the essential oils while the body butter is melting over the stove. If not, blend them drop by drop in a small bowl. Then pour the essential oil blend into the melted body butter, and carefully pour the melted mixture into the glass jars. It will take about 15 minutes to solidify.

FOR KIDS

Substitute:

7 oz (196 g) Luxurious Body Butter (**page 135**)

5 drops neroli

7 drops patchouli

14 drops cedarwood

13 drops gingergrass

LAVENDER'S "ALOE'D TO SLEEP" NIGHTTIME PAIN GEL

Lavender had an active day and was ready to get some sleep, but its muscles were so sore it couldn't rest. This recipe was its solution to both problems.

Use this recipe: to soothe sore muscles so you can get to sleep.

1 oz (28 g) aloe vera gel

5 drops German chamomile

13 drops lavender

DIRECTIONS

Make the blend in a 1 oz (30 ml) glass bottle. Pour the aloe vera into the bottle and add the essential oils.

Shake your blend gently before each use to help distribute the essential oils through the aloe. Massage into achy areas, lie back, and let go.

I recommend making this blend fresh every few weeks.

FOR KIDS

Substitute:

1 oz (28 g) aloe vera gel

3 drops German chamomile

3 drops lavender

Lavender's "Shh, the Baby's Asleep!" Spray

For those nights when cuddles and bedtime stories aren't quite enough for babies and kids, Lavender brings out this relaxing, gentle hydrosol spray to help them sleep.

Use this recipe: to help babies and kids feel relaxed and get to sleep.

2 oz (60 ml) lavender hydrosol

DIRECTIONS

Spritz the lavender hydrosol on blankets, on car seats, and in the crib. You can even spritz some on your own clothes as you hold the baby. (It's okay if it gets on the baby's skin.)

Be sure to check with your supplier about the shelf life of the hydrosol.

Respiration

Essential oils love to be breathed in! It should come as no surprise that so many of them like to help us breathe deeply. The recipes in this chapter are good at clearing congestion, reducing infection, and calming sniffles and coughs.

Some oils stand out from the crowd for their talents in this area (eucalyptus and tea tree come to mind) and their fresh, medicinal, camphoraceous aromas help us identify them as helpful respiratory oils right away. Other respiratory oils have less medicinal aromas, and may smell floral, spicy, citrusy, piney, resinous, or woodsy. You have a wide variety to work with, and it means you can round out your respiratory blends, pairing some of the sharper-smelling oils with some of the softer ones to create scents that really appeal to you.

When it comes to methods of application, inhalation is a big one. You can make diffuser blends, inhalers, and steam blends. Inhaling the steam from a bowl of hot water with a single drop of essential oil in it can feel good when you have a cold or flu. Steaming is a good method to use if you're relaxing at home and have a little time to set up a bowl of hot water several times throughout the day.

Diffusing essential oils is another method of inhalation. A diffuser can fill the whole room with scent, and cleanses the air while helping you breathe more deeply.

Inhalers are convenient. You can carry an aromatherapy inhaler with you in a pocket or bag and use it anytime, anywhere. It doesn't impact the space the way a diffuser does, and it doesn't take the setup time that steaming does. Only you smell the essential oils in an inhaler, and if you have a busy day, you can take it with you. Inhalers are ideal if you have to keep working while you're feeling sick.

Preventive measures can also help you stay healthy. If you're not sniffling at the moment, you can make inhalers to use when you travel or are in places with a lot of people. If you're exposed to someone who is sick, you can do a steam afterward. Another perk to making preventive blends is that they'll already be around if you do come down with something.

This chapter won't overlook using the oils in topical blends, either. Chest rubs and body oils for respiratory support can be especially soothing if you're suffering from physical aches and pains.

As they help you breathe more openly, they also help to expand your emotional sense of openness, optimism, and energy.

Before you make any of the following recipes, be sure to check the shelf lives of your ingredients so you know how long your product will last and any safety concerns for the essential oils.

Eucalyptus's "Get Up and Go" Diffuser Blend

Eucalyptus had a cold and wanted to stay in bed, but it still had a lot to do. This diffuser blend helped it feel energized and focused.

Use this recipe: for clearing congestion and feeling vital enough to go about your day.

3 drops eucalyptus

3 drops cardamom

2 drops rosemary ct. camphor

2 drops lime

DIRECTIONS

Simply drop all the essential oils into the diffuser.

FOR KIDS 💜

Substitute:

2 drops orange

1 drop lavender

1 drop lime

2 drops cedarwood

CEDARWOOD'S "QUIET AND CLEAR" DIFFUSER BLEND

This blend helps Cedarwood stay in touch with a core of quiet strength during a cold. The essential oils help its body rest and its mind feel calm.

Use this recipe: to ease congestion and get some quality, restorative rest.

3 drops rosalina

5 drops cedarwood

2 drops frankincense

DIRECTIONS

Simply drop all the essential oils into the diffuser.

FOR KIDS 💜

Substitute:

3 drops cedarwood

2 drops frankincense

The Conifer Crew's "Allergy Away" Diffuser Blend

Hemlock, Piñon Pine, and Black Spruce combined their strengths for this blend. It continuously calms allergies, so reactions don't have time to set in and cause discomfort.

Use this recipe: for ongoing support to relieve allergies.

4 drops hemlock

1 drop piñon pine

2 drops black spruce

3 drops orange

DIRECTIONS

Simply drop all the essential oils into the diffuser.

FOR KIDS

Substitute:

1 drop hemlock

1 drop piñon pine

1 drop black spruce

2 drops orange

To make these aromatherapy inhalers, follow the directions on **page 132**.

Thyme's "I Don't Have Thyme for Allergies" Inhaler

If you don't have time for allergies, use Thyme for allergies! Thyme ct. linalool made this inhaler to calm allergic reactions in a consistent, comforting way.

Use this recipe: for ongoing support to relieve allergies.

7 drops thyme ct. linalool

4 drops cedarwood

4 drops palo santo

FOR KIDS ♥

Substitute:

3 drops thyme ct. linalool

1 drop cedarwood

1 drop palo santo

Lemon's "Happy and Healthy Trails" Inhaler

Lemon doesn't worry about getting sick when it travels. It takes along this inhaler to prevent sniffles and keep its health strong.

Use this recipe: to keep your spirits bright and your health vital when you're on the road.

4 drops tea tree

3 drops myrtle

6 drops lemon

3 drops juniper

FOR KIDS 🖤

Substitute:

2 drops tea tree

2 drops cedarwood

2 drops lemon

2 drops juniper

BLACK SPRUCE AND HEMLOCK'S "THROAT FRIEND" INHALER

. . . .

Black Spruce and Hemlock don't like coughs and sore throats. They collaborated on this inhaler to make the world a more cough-free place.

. . . .

Use this recipe: to soothe sore throats and respiratory issues that come with an uncomfortable cough.

6 drops black spruce

4 drops hemlock

3 drops myrtle

2 drops thyme ct. linalool

FOR KIDS ♥

Substitute:

2 drops black spruce

2 drops hemlock

1 drop cedarwood

1 drop thyme ct. linalool

LIME AND TEA TREE'S
"FEEL BETTER IN THE MORNING" INHALER

Lime had trouble starting its day when it got sick, so it made this inhaler to help it feel invigorated and clear congestion.

Use this recipe: to start your day feeling healthy, even if you have a cold or flu.

5 drops lime

5 drops tea tree

3 drops lavender

2 drops peppermint

FOR KIDS ♥

Substitute:

2 drops lime

2 drops tea tree

1 drop lavender

Respiration

DIRECTIONS FOR STEAM BLENDS

Make the blend in a 5 ml amber glass bottle. Add the essential oils to the bottle, and then snap the bottle's orifice reducer into place. This makes approximately 1 ml (25 drops) of stock blend.

To do a steam: Fill a glass or ceramic bowl with steamy hot water. Add one drop (just one!) of the stock blend to the water, then close your eyes, lean over the bowl, and inhale the steam. To keep the soothing steam concentrated around your face, drape a towel over your head as you lean over the bowl, making a "towel tent." Be sure to keep your eyes closed and that the steam is not too hot for your skin.

You can steam several times a day to keep breathing clearly, particularly during cold and flu season.

KUNZEA'S "KEEP ON BREATHING" STEAM BLEND

Kunzea loves taking care of people who are sick, but it doesn't want to get sick itself! It uses this steam blend to stay healthy.

Use this recipe: to help prevent yourself from getting sick.

7 drops eucalyptus

13 drops kunzea

8 drops rosemary ct. camphor

7 drops myrtle

FOR KIDS

Steaming can be great for kids over five years old. Use just one drop of the blend below, and have them close their eyes and lean over the bowl to breathe in the warm steam without draping a towel over their head.

6 drops cedarwood

11 drops lavender

8 drops orange

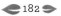

EUCALYPTUS'S "BEST DECONGEST" STEAM BLEND

. . . .

Eucalyptus is a bit of a show-off. It loves to demonstrate how good it is (the best!) at reducing congestion and helping your sinuses feel open instead of clogged.

. . . .

Use this recipe: to clear congestion, mucus, and your sinuses when you're stuffed up, sniffly, or sneezy.

12 drops eucalyptus

9 drops thyme ct. linalool

8 drops tea tree

7 drops juniper

FOR KIDS 🖤

Steaming can be great for kids over five years old. Use just one drop of the blend below, and have them close their eyes and lean over the bowl to breathe in the warm steam without draping a towel over their head.

12 drops cedarwood

9 drops thyme ct. linalool

8 drops tea tree

7 drops juniper

Saro's "Seriously Soothing" Chest Rub

Saro partnered with its gentle friends Myrrh and Thyme ct. linalool to make this chest rub to support easy breathing and be considerate of skin at the same time.

Use this recipe: as a chest rub to help you breathe deeply and easily.

7 oz (196 g) Luxurious Body Butter (**page 135**)

38 drops saro

23 drops myrrh

18 drops juniper

26 drops thyme ct. linalool

DIRECTIONS

Use four 2 oz (60 ml) glass jars when making the Luxurious Body Butter on **page 135**. If you have a graduated cylinder, you can measure out the essential oils while the body butter is melting over the stove. If not, blend them drop by drop in a small bowl. Then pour the essential oil blend into the melted body butter, and carefully pour the melted mixture into the glass jars.

When the blend cools, you can rub it on your chest, lie back, relax, and breathe deeply.

FOR KIDS ♥

Substitute:

7 oz (196 g) Luxurious Body Butter (**page 135**)

16 drops cedarwood

8 drops myrrh

8 drops juniper

10 drops thyme ct. linalool

MYRRH'S "SPRUCE ME UP" RESPIRATORY OIL

Myrrh made this oil to remind you that when you have a respiratory issue, your whole body needs TLC—not only your nose and throat.

Use this recipe: as an allover body oil to ease aches and pains that come along with respiratory discomfort.

1 oz (30 ml) trauma oil

2 drops basil ct. linalool

3 drops piñon pine

5 drops black spruce

5 drops myrrh

DIRECTIONS

Make the blend in a 1 oz (30 ml) glass bottle. Pour the trauma oil into the bottle, and add the essential oils.

FOR KIDS 💛

Substitute:

1 oz (30 ml) trauma oil

1 drop basil ct. linalool

1 drop piñon pine

2 drops black spruce

2 drops myrrh

Respiration

KUNZEA AND CEDARWOOD'S "SKIN SO SOOTHED" ALLERGY OIL

Kunzea and Cedarwood know that allergens can irritate your skin as much as your nose. Their moisturizing allergy oil lets your body truly absorb their support to reduce reactions.

Use this recipe: as an allover moisturizer that can help calm allergies.

1 oz (30 ml) jojoba

8 drops kunzea

8 drops cedarwood

DIRECTIONS

Make the blend in a 1 oz (30 ml) glass roller-top bottle. Pour the jojoba into the bottle, add the essential oils, and then snap the roller-top into place.

FOR KIDS

Substitute:

1 oz (30 ml) jojoba

3 drops lavender

3 drops cedarwood

Juniper's "My Body Feels Better All Over" Butter

Juniper's friends came down with a cold and felt too sore and achy (not to mention sniffly) to have fun. It created this body butter to help them feel better fast.

Use this recipe: to ease aches and pains, and reduce infections when you're sick.

7 oz (196 g) Luxurious Body Butter (**page 135**)

32 drops piñon pine

27 drops black spruce

32 drops juniper

17 drops hemlock

DIRECTIONS

Use four 2 oz (60 ml) glass jars when making the Luxurious Body Butter on **page 135**. If you have a graduated cylinder, you can measure out the essential oils while the body butter is melting over the stove. If not, blend them drop by drop in a small bowl. Then pour the essential oil blend into the melted body butter, and carefully pour the melted mixture into the glass jars.

FOR KIDS ♡

Substitute:

7 oz (196 g) Luxurious Body Butter (**page 135**)

9 drops piñon pine

13 drops hemlock

7 drops juniper

13 drops Roman chamomile

Respiration

Rosalina's "Soothing Muscle Soak" Bath Salts

Sore muscles? Sniffles? Stuffed up? Not when Rosalina's around! Let Rosalina fill the bathtub with warm water and muscle-relaxing bath salt for you.

Use this recipe: to soothe achy muscles and reduce congestion.

2 oz (56 g) salt

1 teaspoon (5 ml) vanilla-infused jojoba

2 drops rosalina

3 drops lavender

DIRECTIONS

Use a 2 oz (60 ml) glass jar for this blend.

Put the salt into the jar. Blend the jojoba and essential oils in a separate bowl before adding to the salt. Stir with a glass stirring rod or the handle of a stainless-steel spoon.

Each recipe makes enough for one bath. If you love it, you can make more and store it in a glass jar. The jojoba provides a skin-nourishing carrier to distribute the essential oils.

Pay attention to your skin's responses when using essential oils in a bath. What's comfortable for you may be different from what's comfortable for other people. You may want more jojoba, less essential oil, or different essential oils from the ones in the recipe.

I suggest using about five drops of essential oil total in a warm bath.

I recommend making this blend fresh every few weeks.

FOR KIDS ♡

Substitute:

2 oz (56 g) salt

1 teaspoon (5 ml) jojoba

2 drops cedarwood

1 drop lavender

Hemlock's "Wake Up and Smile" Shower Gel

Hemlock wants you to start the day with a smile and a deep breath, even when you have a cold. A warm, steamy shower with this blend can help that happen.

Use this recipe: as a morning shower gel that cleanses skin and opens your breath.

1 oz (28 g) aloe vera gel

2 drops gingergrass

3 drops yuzu

3 drops hemlock

3 drops spike lavender

DIRECTIONS

Make the blend in a 1 oz (30 ml) flip-top bottle. Pour the aloe into the bottle and add the essential oils.

Shake the blend gently before each use to help distribute the essential oils through the aloe.

I recommend making this blend fresh every few weeks.

FOR KIDS ♥

Substitute:

1 oz (28 g) aloe vera gel

1 drop gingergrass

2 drops yuzu

1 drop hemlock

2 drops cedarwood

Rosemary's "Really Clean, Really Healthy" Foam Soap

Keeping things clean is Rosemary's favorite way of preventing infections from spreading. It made this natural foam soap so you don't have to use commercial soaps that might irritate your skin.

Use this recipe: to wash your hands and reduce infections.

1.4 oz (40 ml) castile soap

1 teaspoon (5 g) aloe vera gel

6 drops thyme ct. linalool

8 drops bergamot mint

6 drops saro

10 drops rosemary ct. camphor

DIRECTIONS

Use a 50 ml foam soap pump bottle. There will be extra space in the top of the bottle to allow room for the pump. Pour the castile soap and aloe into the bottle, and then add the essential oils.

I recommend making this blend fresh every few weeks.

FOR KIDS

Substitute:

1.4 oz (40 ml) castile soap

1 teaspoon (5 g) aloe vera gel

4 drops bergamot mint

3 drops thyme ct. linalool

5 drops lavender

2 drops orange

Palmarosa's
"Ultrarelaxing Allergy-Reducing"
Linen Spray

When allergies interrupted Palmarosa's sleep, it got up and made this linen spray. The blend is relaxing *and* allergy-reducing.

Use this recipe: to relax, calm allergic reactions, and reduce allergens that might be on your linens (such as dust mites).

1 oz (30 ml) frankincense hydrosol

9 drops palmarosa

4 drops frankincense

5 drops saro

DIRECTIONS

Use a 1 oz (30 ml) glass bottle for this blend. Combine all the ingredients in the bottle, give it a shake, and spritz your sheets and underneath your pillowcases with it.

I recommend making this blend fresh every few weeks.

FOR KIDS ♥

Substitute:

1 oz (30 ml) frankincense hydrosol

4 drops palmarosa

2 drops frankincense

Respiration

These aloe-based hand cleansers are made without chemical ingredients that might cause dryness or irritation.

DIRECTIONS FOR HAND CLEANSERS

Use a 1 oz (30 ml) PET plastic flip-top bottle. Put the aloe vera gel and essential oils into the bottle, give it a shake, and use it as an on-the-go hand cleanser.

Shake your blend gently before each use to help distribute the essential oils through the aloe.

I recommend making these blends fresh every few weeks.

THYME'S "EVERYTHING BUT THE SINK" HAND CLEANSER

Thyme loves washing its hands frequently to reduce infections. This recipe has everything it needs (but the sink!) to cleanse and care for its hands while it's running around town.

Use this recipe: to cleanse your hands on the go.

1 oz (28 g) aloe vera gel

8 drops thyme ct. linalool

5 drops lemon

5 drops tea tree

FOR KIDS ♡

Substitute:

1 oz (28 g) aloe vera gel

3 drops thyme ct. linalool

1 drop lemon

2 drop tea tree

Piñon Pine's "Clean in the Woods" Hand Cleanser

Piñon Pine loves spending time in nature, but that doesn't mean it likes to get dirty. It takes along this hand cleanser, particularly for cleaning up before meals.

Use this recipe: to cleanse your hands on the go.

1 oz (28 g) aloe vera gel

10 drops piñon pine

8 drops rosalina

FOR KIDS

Substitute:

1 oz (28 g) aloe vera gel

5 drops piñon pine

4 drops cedarwood

Digestion

One of the most profound early experiences I had with essential oils was when I used a drop of Roman chamomile in a little jojoba to relieve tension in my belly. I could not believe how quickly and effectively the Roman chamomile worked. It was gentle, yet powerful. I felt the tension quickly dissipate from my belly. This was one of the experiences that encouraged me to study aromatherapy in depth.

Stress and tension are only a few issues that can cause stomach discomfort. A few others are indigestion, gas, nausea, motion sickness, cramps, and even wearing a belt that's a little too tight. Sometimes you know what the cause is, while other times you may not be quite sure why your belly hurts.

There are many causes of stomach discomfort, and you can use many of the same essential oils for all of them. You don't need to collect different oils for each kind of stomach issue. This is such a relief, especially if you don't know what's causing the discomfort.

The essential oils in these recipes are known for calming muscle spasms, easing tension, reducing inflammation, and soothing pain. Some of the belly-friendly oils are more "energizing," such as cardamom and lime, while others are more relaxing, such as Roman chamomile. Once you get a feel for the kinds of oils that work for you, you can get creative. Maybe you'll prefer the "antispasmodic" oils, or the oils known for pain relief. Maybe the citruses or the spices will be your belly's best friends.

Topical creams and oils applied to your belly and lower back can feel surprisingly soothing as they calm the muscles in and around your abdomen, and inhalers are remarkably helpful for issues like nausea and motion sickness. In some cases, you may want to combine a topical blend with an inhaler to address the discomfort from multiple angles.

Finding the right belly blend for you can really set you at ease. These recipes will give you a lot of options and ideas to work with.

Before you make any of the following recipes, be sure to check the shelf lives of your ingredients so you know how long your product will last, and any safety concerns for the essential oils.

Orange's "Spiked" Belly Butter

. . . .

Orange made a big meal for friends and accidentally ate too much itself. Fortunately Spikenard brought this belly butter—so comforting after a big, delicious meal!

. . . .

Use this recipe: to soothe a tight and expanded belly after a big meal.

7 oz (196 g) Luxurious Body Butter (**page 135**)

14 drops ginger

21 drops Roman chamomile

14 drops spikenard

35 drops orange

DIRECTIONS

Use four 2 oz (60 ml) glass jars when making the Luxurious Body Butter (**page 135**).

Rub the belly butter on your belly and low back before or after eating (or both!), and take a moment to breath and relax.

FOR KIDS 💙

Substitute:

7 oz (196 g) Luxurious Body Butter (**page 135**)

7 drops ginger

10 drops Roman chamomile

7 drops spikenard

17 drops orange

Roman Chamomile's "Cramp Calm" Cream

Basil had indigestion, Cardamom had belly cramps, and Lime felt nervous about publishing its new recipe book. Roman Chamomile soothed each of their stomachs with one batch of this Cramp Calm Cream.

Use this recipe: to calm belly cramps.

7 oz (196 g) Luxurious Body Butter (**page 135**)

21 drops cardamom

14 drops basil ct. linalool

21 drops lime

28 drops Roman chamomile

DIRECTIONS

Use four 2 oz (60 ml) glass jars when making the Luxurious Body Butter (**page 135**). If you have a graduated cylinder, you can measure out the essential oils while the body butter is melting over the stove. If not, blend them drop by drop in a small bowl. Then pour the essential oil blend into the melted body butter, stir gently with a glass stirring stick or the handle of a stainless-steel spoon, and carefully pour the melted mixture into the glass jars.

Once the Cramp Calm Cream has cooled and solidified, rub it on your belly and low back so your stomach (and you) can actually relax.

FOR KIDS

Substitute:

7 oz (196 g) Luxurious Body Butter (**page 135**)

10 drops orange

7 drops basil ct. linalool

10 drops lime

14 drops Roman chamomile

To make these aromatherapy inhalers, follow the directions on **page 132**.

BASIL'S "PAT YOUR HEAD AND RUB YOUR BELLY" INHALER

Sometimes Basil has muscle tension in multiple places at once, such as in its belly and head. Taking deep breaths of this inhaler helps Basil release that stress and relax.

Use this recipe: to ease an upset stomach and a headache at the same time.

4 drops peppermint

5 drops bergamot mint

7 drops basil ct. linalool

FOR KIDS 💜

Substitute:

2 drops orange

2 drops bergamot mint

3 drops basil ct. linalool

Myrtle's
"I've Got Places to Go!"
Nausea Inhaler

When Myrtle goes traveling, it wants to experience adventure, not nausea. It uses this inhaler to both relieve nausea and help prevent it altogether.

Use this recipe: to reduce nausea and support your health while you're traveling.

4 drops ginger

5 drops orange

6 drops myrtle

FOR KIDS ♥

Substitute:

2 drops ginger

2 drops orange

3 drops lavender

Bergamot Mint's "Out on the Town or in for the Night" Nausea Inhaler

Sometimes Bergamot Mint wants to go out and have fun. Sometimes it wants to stay in and relax with a good book. Either way, it uses this inhaler when nausea interrupts its plans.

Use this recipe: for calming nausea and feeling uplifted.

4 drops peppermint

5 drops orange

6 drops bergamot mint

FOR KIDS 💚

Substitute:

2 drops cedarwood

2 drops orange

3 drops bergamot mint

Peppermint and Yuzu's "Too Much Food to Move" Belly Oil

Peppermint took Yuzu out for a big dinner, but then they both felt too full to go dancing. Fortunately Peppermint brought along this belly oil, and they both danced the night way!

Use this recipe: when you've eaten too much, have belly cramps, and feel like you can't move.

1 oz (30 ml) jojoba

4 drops peppermint

2 drops lime

4 drops yuzu

2 drops bergamot mint

DIRECTIONS

Make the blend in a 1 oz (30 ml) glass bottle. Pour the jojoba into the bottle and add the essential oils drop by drop.

Massage into your belly and low back after you've eaten a big meal. You can also use it before you eat to help make sure you keep feeling good after the last bite.

FOR KIDS

Substitute:

1 oz (30 ml) jojoba

2 drops orange

1 drop lime

2 drops yuzu

1 drop bergamot mint

LIME'S "COMFY BELLY, OPEN HEART" OIL

Lime's friends came in from out of town for dinner, but all that traveling left them a little too tense to enjoy their meal. Lime passed around this soothing belly oil, and everyone relaxed and ate their fill.

Use this recipe: to soothe emotional and physical tension that resides in your belly.

1 oz (30 ml) jojoba

2 drops ylang ylang

6 drops bergamot mint

2 drops ginger

6 drops lime

DIRECTIONS

Make the blend in a 1 oz (30 ml) glass bottle. Pour the jojoba into the bottle, and add the essential oils.

FOR KIDS

Substitute:

1 oz (30 ml) jojoba

1 drop ylang ylang

2 drops bergamot mint

1 drop ginger

2 drops lime

Digestion

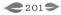

Two Bath Salt Blends

DIRECTIONS FOR BATH SALTS

Use a 2 oz (60 ml) glass jar for this blend.

Put the salt into the jar. Blend the jojoba and essential oils in a separate bowl before adding to the salt. Stir with a glass stirring rod or the handle of a stainless-steel spoon. Each recipe makes enough for one bath. If you love it, you can make more and store it in a glass jar. The jojoba provides a skin-nourishing carrier to distribute the essential oils.

Pay attention to your skin's responses when using essential oils in a bath. What's comfortable for you may be different from what's comfortable for other people. You may want more jojoba, less essential oil, or different essential oils from the ones in the recipes.

I suggest using about five drops of essential oil total in a bath.

I recommend making these blends fresh every few weeks.

ROMAN CHAMOMILE'S "DINNER AND A WARM BATH" SALTS

Roman Chamomile uses this bath salt to help it release tension in its belly and all over its body. It's perfect after a long day and a big dinner.

Use this recipe: to help you digest and relax during a warm bath.

2 oz (56 g) salt

1 teaspoon (5 ml) jojoba

2 drops yuzu

3 drops Roman chamomile

FOR KIDS 🖤

Substitute: 2 oz (56 g) salt, 1 teaspoon (5 ml) jojoba, 1 drop yuzu, 2 drops Roman chamomile

ORANGE'S "AFTER-TREAT RETREAT" BATH SALT

Orange's favorite follow-up to dinner is dessert. Its favorite follow-up to dessert is a cup of tea. Its favorite follow-up to a full belly is a warm bath to help it feel calm and comfortable.

Use this recipe: to rest and digest after you've had a delicious meal (and dessert!).

2 oz (56 g) salt

1 teaspoon (5 ml) jojoba

2 drops orange

3 drops spikenard

FOR KIDS 🖤

Substitute:

2 oz (56 g) salt

1 teaspoon (5 ml) jojoba

1 drop orange

2 drops spikenard

Bergamot Mint's "Dinner in an Orchard" Diffuser Blend

Bergamot Mint loves having dinner in its backyard orchard. When the weather's rainy or cold, it diffuses this essential oil blend to create the same atmosphere indoors.

Use this recipe: to create a relaxing environment that makes it easy to digest a good meal.

5 drops bergamot mint

1 drop orange

2 drops lime

2 drops yuzu

DIRECTIONS

Simply drop the essential oils into the diffuser.

FOR KIDS

Substitute:

3 drops bergamot mint

1 drop orange

1 drop yuzu

Yuzu's "Clean Up before You Eat Up" Foam Hand Soap

Does washing its hands before dinner help Yuzu digest its meal more easily? Not really. But it does reduce Yuzu's chances of getting sick, and this soap makes its hands smell amazing.

Use this recipe: to clean your hands before and after dinner.

1.4 oz (40 ml) castile soap

1 teaspoon (5 g) aloe vera gel

5 drops peppermint

8 drops yuzu

7 drops lime

DIRECTIONS

Use a 50 ml foam soap pump bottle. There will be extra space at the top of the bottle to allow room for the pump.

I recommend making this blend fresh every few weeks.

FOR KIDS

Substitute:

1.4 oz (40 ml) castile soap

1 teaspoon (5 g) aloe vera gel

2 drops orange

4 drops yuzu

3 drops lime

Pain Relief

You know that feeling good can support your well-being, but what if you've been injured or are ill? It's not easy to feel good if you're laid up in recovery with a broken leg or if you have a chronic condition that causes daily discomfort. At times like these, the effects that essential oils can have on your mind and heart—and yes, also on your body—can offer a lot of support.

Simply surrounding yourself with aromas you love can help keep your mind calm and your heart uplifted. It is a good way to care for yourself during times when you're susceptible to becoming overwhelmed, afraid, or anxious. Staying relaxed may be more difficult when you're in pain, but it's just as important, if not more so. If you can relax, it helps to reduce stress levels in your body and create more room for healing to take place.

Many "healing" essential oils like to combine their special talents for reducing inflammation and easing pain with their emotional qualities. So if you make an oil for a sprained ankle, it can help to support your healing and keep you feeling happy. If you make a joint salve for painful knees at night, it can also help you rest and sleep peacefully. You can make your blend with ingredients that won't get all over your sheets!

It's a good idea to consider how long you'll need a pain relief blend before you make it. Some of the recipes in this chapter are best used for "acute" symptoms that don't last very long, such as a sprained ankle or an infection. These blends are often made with higher concentrations of essential oils. Other recipes are helpful for conditions that need ongoing support over longer periods of time, such as chronic joint inflammation. These recipes use lower concentrations of the oils, and they also include skin-nourishing ingredients that won't cause irritation if you use them over a long period of time.

Unless your discomfort has a chronic nature, you may not know you need a pain relief blend until you actually need it, when the last thing you might feel like doing is making an aromatherapy blend! That said, you can sometimes plan ahead and anticipate potential needs. If you enjoy running, make a few blends for sore, tense muscles or sprained ankles to have on hand. If you're going camping, make a few itch sticks and emergency blends ahead of time to soothe cuts and scrapes.

Recovering from a chronic issue or injury always takes its own course. It's not something you can control. You can, however, put yourself in a position to feel better and encourage the healing process. Before you make any of the following recipes, be sure to check the shelf lives of your ingredients so you know how long your product will last, and any safety concerns for the essential oils. Also, pay attention to the directions for using each recipe, and use only blends specifically created for use on cuts or scrapes to apply to broken skin.

Spike Lavender's "Sore Muscle Miracle" Oil

Spike Lavender loves to run, jump, swim, hike, climb mountains, and dance its heart out! After a day full of fun, it massages its sore muscles with this blend.

Use this recipe: to soothe sore muscles during massage.

1 oz (30 ml) trauma oil

7 drops spike lavender

4 drops black spruce

4 drops myrtle

3 drops ginger

DIRECTIONS

Make the blend in a 1 oz (30 ml) glass bottle. Pour the trauma oil into the bottle and add the essential oils.

FOR KIDS

Substitute:

1 oz (30 ml) trauma oil

3 drops lavender

2 drops black spruce

1 drop orange

GINGERGRASS'S "EASE UP" MUSCLE OIL

Gingergrass is a master of strong, flexible, happy muscles. It does yoga every day, and if its muscles feel sore afterward, it uses this massage oil to care for them.

Use this recipe: to ease tight, painful muscles and encourage flexibility.

1 oz (30 ml) trauma oil

8 drops gingergrass

4 drops saro

3 drops cardamom

2 drops geranium

DIRECTIONS

Make the blend in a 1 oz (30 ml) glass bottle. Pour the trauma oil into the bottle and add the essential oils.

FOR KIDS

Substitute:

1 oz (30 ml) trauma oil

3 drops gingergrass

1 drop lavender

1 drop cedarwood

1 drop geranium

Juniper's "Jumping for Joy" Joint Gel

Many people come to Juniper when their joints feel inflamed and inflexible. Juniper massages their joints with this gel until they're jumping for joy!

Use this recipe: to soothe painful and swollen joints.

1 oz (28 g) aloe vera gel

6 drops juniper

4 drops German chamomile

4 drops palmarosa

4 drops lemon

DIRECTIONS

Make the blend in a 1 oz (30 ml) glass bottle. Pour the aloe vera gel into the bottle and add the essential oils.

Shake the blend gently before each use to help distribute the essential oils through the aloe.

I recommend making this blend fresh every few weeks.

FOR KIDS 💙

Substitute:

1 oz (28 g) aloe vera gel

3 drops juniper

1 drop German chamomile

1 drop palmarosa

1 drop lemon

Cardamom's "4/9 Joint Care" Oil

Cardamom, Rosemary ct. camphor, Geranium, and Peppermint all had an equal role in making this blend ... and they're all talented at soothing pain, reducing chronic swelling, and encouraging circulation.

Use this recipe: to encourage circulation, reduce inflammation, and bring relief to painful joints.

2 oz (60 ml) arnica oil

9 drops cardamom

9 drops rosemary ct. camphor

9 drops geranium

9 drops peppermint

DIRECTIONS

Make the blend in a 2 oz (60 ml) glass bottle. Pour the arnica oil into the bottle and add the essential oils. Massage into swollen joints.

FOR KIDS

You can call this "3/4 Joint Care for Kids." Substitute:

2 oz (60 ml) arnica oil

4 drops cedarwood

4 drops orange

4 drops geranium

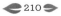

HEMLOCK'S "I FEEL SWELL" OIL

Hemlock made this oil to encourage circulation, reduce inflammation, and feel cool on warm areas. After using this oil, you'll feel swell instead of swollen.

Use this recipe: to massage away swelling and to warm up cold, tight joints.

2 oz (60 ml) trauma oil

15 drops hemlock

8 drops Roman chamomile

8 drops German chamomile

5 drops lemon

DIRECTIONS

Make the blend in a 0.35 oz (10 ml) glass bottle. Pour the trauma oil into the bottle and add the essential oils. Massage into painful, swollen areas.

FOR KIDS 💙

Substitute:

2 oz (60 ml) trauma oil

4 drops hemlock

3 drops Roman chamomile

3 drops German chamomile

2 drops lemon

Roman Chamomile's "Extra Helpful" Headache and Belly Oil

. . . .

When Roman Chamomile's friends have headaches or nausea, it takes them on relaxing riverboat tours. If they still need a little extra help, Roman Chamomile applies this soothing oil to their neck, belly, and chest.

. . . .

Use this recipe: to relieve a headache accompanied by nausea.

0.35 oz (10 ml) trauma oil

2 drops Roman chamomile

2 drops frankincense

2 drops ginger

DIRECTIONS

Make the blend in a 0.35 oz (10 ml) glass roller-top bottle. Pour the trauma oil into the bottle, add the essential oils, then snap the roller-top into place. Apply to the neck, belly, and chest.

FOR KIDS ♡

Substitute:

0.35 oz (10 ml) trauma oil

1 drop Roman chamomile

1 drop frankincense

1 drop ginger

Rosemary's "Easy Focus" Headache Inhaler

Rosemary made this inhaler when it studied too long and developed a tension headache. The inhaler eases pain and helps Rosemary keep on concentrating.

Use this recipe: to relieve a tension headache and encourage mental focus.

9 drops rosemary ct. camphor

3 drops spike lavender

3 drops basil ct. linalool

FOR KIDS

Substitute:

4 drops orange

1 drop lavender

1 drop basil ct. linalool

Piñon Pine's
"Minus the Sinus Headache"
Inhaler

Piñon Pine was having a fantastic day until a sinus headache set in. It added a few essential oils to an inhaler and subtracted the tension and pressure from its sinuses.

Use this recipe: to ease headaches and pressure in your sinus cavity.

8 drops piñon pine

2 drops hemlock

5 drops kunzea

FOR KIDS ♥

Substitute:

3 drops piñon pine

1 drop hemlock

2 drops cedarwood

HELICHRYSUM'S "NO MORE BLACK-AND-BLUES" BRUISE OIL

When friends get bruises and feel sad, Helichrysum gives them this healing blend. It clears up bruises almost as quickly as it clears up the blues!

Use this recipe: to help bruises heal quickly.

1 oz (30 ml) trauma oil

9 drops helichrysum

5 drops lavender

4 drops German chamomile

DIRECTIONS

Make the blend in a 1 oz (30 ml) glass bottle. Pour the trauma oil into the bottle and add the essential oils. Apply gently to the bruise as often as needed until the bruise disappears.

FOR KIDS

Substitute:

1 oz (30 ml) trauma oil

4 drops helichrysum

1 drop lavender

1 drop German chamomile

Pain Relief

LAVENDER'S "BAND-AID IN A BOTTLE" GEL

Lavender keeps a bottle of this blend within reach in case someone gets a cut or scrape. Lavender washes the area, applies this gel, and its mind feels at ease knowing the cut is clean and will heal well.

Use this recipe: to help small cuts and scrapes heal more quickly.

1 oz (28 g) aloe vera gel

7 drops frankincense

3 drops lavender

5 drops cedarwood

3 drops helichrysum

DIRECTIONS

Make the blend in a 1 oz (30 ml) glass bottle. Pour the aloe vera into the bottle and add the essential oils.

Shake the blend gently before each use to help distribute the essential oils through the aloe. Cleanse the wound, and then gently apply the blend directly to the cut or scrape.

I recommend making this blend fresh every few weeks.

FOR KIDS 💜

Substitute:

1 oz (28 g) aloe vera gel

2 drops frankincense

1 drop lavender

2 drops cedarwood

1 drop helichrysum

German Chamomile's "Ouch Away" Hydrosol Spray

When kids fall down and get scraped knees, they run to German Chamomile and ask for its famous "Ouch Away" spray. A little spray can ease a lot of pain, and German Chamomile makes it without any essential oils.

Use this recipe: to soothe pain on a fresh cut, scrape, or bruise.

2 oz (60 ml) German chamomile hydrosol

1 oz (30 ml) tea tree hydrosol

1 oz (30 ml) vetiver hydrosol

DIRECTIONS

Simply blend the hydrosols in a 4 oz (120 ml) glass spray bottle. Gently spray the blend directly on a cut or scrape.

I recommend making this blend fresh every few weeks.

FOR KIDS 💜

The version for kids is the same as the one for grown-ups.

Helichrysum's "S.O.S." Pain Relief Oil

Acute injuries like sprains or muscle strains call for immediate help. Helichrysum responds right away to relieve pain and calm inflammation with this soothing oil.

Use this recipe: to ease pain and calm your emotions after an acute injury, such as a sprain.

1 oz (30 ml) trauma oil

8 drops helichrysum

4 drops neroli

6 drops palmarosa

DIRECTIONS

Make the blend in a 1 oz (30 ml) glass bottle. Pour the trauma oil into the bottle and add the essential oils.

FOR KIDS

Substitute:

1 oz (30 ml) trauma oil

3 drops helichrysum

1 drops neroli

2 drops palmarosa

Trauma Oil's "Total Care" Scar Oil

Trauma oil knows that scars are usually around for a long term. That's why it made a scar oil that's deeply nourishing for skin and deeply healing for scars.

Use this recipe: to reduce the appearance of scars and nourish the surrounding skin.

1 oz (30 ml) trauma oil

3 drops geranium

6 drops lavender

6 drops helichrysum

3 drops frankincense

DIRECTIONS

Make the blend in a 1 oz (30 ml) glass bottle. Pour the trauma oil into the bottle and add the essential oils. Apply to the scar and the surrounding area as often as needed.

FOR KIDS

Substitute:

1 oz (30 ml) trauma oil

1 drop geranium

2 drops lavender

2 drops helichrysum

1 drop frankincense

Lavender's "Easy Earache Relief" Oil

Lavender understands that no pain is easy to handle, but earaches can be especially painful. This blend helps reduce the pain and relax muscles in the surrounding area.

Use this recipe: to relieve the pain of earaches.

1 oz (30 ml) trauma oil

7 drops lavender

6 drops eucalyptus

2 drops juniper

3 drops palo santo

DIRECTIONS

Make the blend in a 1 oz (30 ml) glass roller-top bottle. Pour the trauma oil into the bottle and add the essential oils.

Roll gently behind your ear and onto your neck (the same side as the hurt ear). Essential oils must *never* be used inside the ears.

FOR KIDS

Substitute:

1 oz (30 ml) trauma oil

3 drops lavender

1 drop cedarwood

1 drop juniper

1 drop palo santo

Roman Chamomile's
"I Fell Down and I Hurt All Over!"
Bath Salt

Roman Chamomile slipped and fell, and later it felt sore all over. A warm bath with this blend helped relax its muscles, reduce swelling, and comforted Roman Chamomile's heart.

Use this recipe: to ease pain and feel better after you've been injured.

2 oz (56 g) salt

1 teaspoon (5 ml) vanilla-infused jojoba

3 drops Roman chamomile

2 drops frankincense

1 drop rose

DIRECTIONS

Use a 2 oz (60 ml) glass jar for this blend.

Put the salt into the jar. Blend the jojoba and essential oils in a separate bowl before adding to the salt. Stir with a glass stirring rod or the handle of a stainless-steel spoon.

This recipe makes enough for one bath. If you love it, you can make more and store it in a glass jar. The jojoba is a nice addition, providing a skin-nourishing carrier to distribute the essential oils.

I recommend making this blend fresh every few weeks.

FOR KIDS

Substitute:

2 oz (56 g) salt

1 teaspoon (5 ml) vanilla-infused jojoba

2 drops Roman chamomile

1 drop frankincense

1 drop rose

Pain Relief

Meditation and Contemplation

There's something about changing the aroma of a space that can change your entire experience of the space . . . and sometimes your experience of yourself.

Maybe that's why many people throughout history have used aromatherapy in sacred contexts, for rituals and ceremonies. It can help shift our minds into deeper states of meditation, concentration, inner contemplation, and peace.

Incense and oils can be used when you want to deeply connect with yourself. If you're journaling, they can help you access deeper levels of self-reflection. If you're getting a massage, they can help your mind release worry and relax. If you're practicing yoga, they can help you stay centered and uplifted. This chapter is called "Meditation and Contemplation," but you really can use these blends for any personal practice.

There are recipes to make your own loose incense with raw resins, such as frankincense and myrrh, and you can customize them with ingredients like wood chips, dried herbs, or flowers. There are also diffuser blends and body oils in this chapter.

Many of the essential oils in these recipes have resinous, woody, or earthy aromas. Base notes are popular in blends for meditation because they have the ability to ground you in the present moment, helping you feel more connected with your body and surroundings. I love the idea that "grounding is the first step toward soaring"! Floral aromas add notes of beauty and harmony, while lighter notes such as the citruses can help you feel uplifted as you focus your mind.

As with most aromatherapy recipes, it all depends on what you want to experience! Have fun with these blends.

Before you make any of the following recipes, be sure to check the shelf lives of your ingredients so you know how long your product will last, and any safety considerations for the essential oils.

Frankincense's
"Exotic Hypnotic" Diffuser Blend

Frankincense visited its friend Ylang Ylang in Madagascar, and was deeply inspired by the exotic and peaceful location. It made this diffuser blend to re-create that atmosphere.

Use this recipe: to create an exotic aroma and a relaxing atmosphere.

8 drops frankincense

2 drops ylang ylang

DIRECTIONS

Simply drop the essential oils into the diffuser.

FOR KIDS 🖤

Substitute:

4 drops frankincense

1 drop ylang ylang

Bergamot Mint's
"Go with the Glow" Diffuser Blend

Bergamot Mint diffuses this blend in its yoga classes to feel energized and centered, and to get that "yoga glow."

Use this recipe: to feel energized and centered during yoga, tai chi, or another movement practice.

4 drops gingergrass

4 drops bergamot mint

2 drops lavender

DIRECTIONS

Simply drop the essential oils into the diffuser.

FOR KIDS 🖤

Substitute:

2 drops gingergrass

2 drops bergamot mint

1 drop lavender

Juniper's
"Breathe In Inspiration" Diffuser Blend

Juniper created this blend because it loves environments that are full of vibrant energy and the feeling that anything is possible.

Use this recipe: to get your energy flowing and feel uplifted.

3 drops juniper

3 drops piñon pine

3 drops lemon

DIRECTIONS

Simply drop the essential oils into the diffuser.

FOR KIDS

Substitute:

1 drop juniper

2 drops piñon pine

2 drops lemon

Patchouli and Myrrh's "Peace on the Go" Inhaler

Patchouli and Myrrh love to "commit random acts of peace," including giving flowers to others and handing out these inhalers to help people feel calm if their schedules are busy.

Use this recipe: to feel peaceful in the middle of a busy day.

6 drops patchouli

6 drops myrrh

1 drop rose

2 drops Roman chamomile

DIRECTIONS

Add the essential oil drops to the cotton component of an aromatherapy inhaler.

FOR KIDS

Substitute:

3 drops patchouli

3 drops myrrh

1 drop rose

1 drop Roman chamomile

Bergamot Mint's "Pocket of Peace" Inhaler

Bergamot Mint carries this inhaler in its pocket to use anytime it wants to take a few minutes to breathe in an aroma it loves. It's like having a pocket of peace and relaxation!

Use this recipe: to calm your nervous system and uplift your heart.

6 drops bergamot mint

3 drops spikenard

3 drops cedarwood

3 drops frankincense

DIRECTIONS

Add the essential oil drops to the cotton component of an aromatherapy inhaler.

FOR KIDS ♡

Substitute:

3 drops bergamot mint

1 drop spikenard

1 drop cedarwood

1 drop frankincense

Frankincense's "Awake and Attentive" Room and Body Spritz

. . . .

Frankincense is a master of meditation. It's good at focusing its mind even in unlikely situations, such as when it's very tired but still has some work to complete.

. . . .

Use this recipe: to feel focused and alert when you're tired but still have a lot to do.

3 oz (90 ml) frankincense hydrosol

1 oz (30 ml) peppermint hydrosol

DIRECTIONS

Simply blend the hydrosols in a 4 oz (120 ml) glass spray bottle.

I recommend making this blend fresh every few weeks.

FOR KIDS ♥

The blend for kids is the same as the one for grown-ups.

Peppermint's
"Pep Your Engines" Car Spritz

Peppermint loves road trips! It can drive for a long time without getting tired. How does it keep its energy up? It sprays this fresh, revitalizing car spritz all around its car and on the back of the neck.

Use this recipe: to stay energized, alert, and enthusiastic on long road trips, especially during hot days.

4 oz (120 ml) peppermint hydrosol

DIRECTIONS

Simply pour the hydrosol in a 4 oz (120 ml) glass spray bottle.

Be sure to check with your supplier about the shelf life of your hydrosol. This blend may not be right for cars with leather upholstery.

FOR KIDS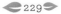

The blend for kids is the same as the one for grown-ups.

Meditation and Contemplation

Opopanax's
"Ancient Princess" Perfume Balm

Opopanax developed this perfume on an archaeological dig in the palace of an ancient princess. It wore its new perfume and noticed that it was able to settle into its work more deeply.

Use this recipe: as a perfume that makes you smell sweet and helps you feel grounded.

½ oz (15 ml) neroli-infused jojoba

1½ oz (42 g) beeswax

18 drops opopanax

8 drops palo santo

10 drops neroli

DIRECTIONS

Make the blend in a 2 oz (60 ml) glass jar.

Set up the Stovetop Melting Method (**pages 133–134**). Melt the beeswax in the Pyrex measuring cup. Add the neroli-infused jojoba. When the beeswax and jojoba are melted together, remove the blend from the heat and add the essential oils. Pour the blend into the jar and wait for it to cool (about 15 minutes).

FOR KIDS

Substitute:

½ oz (15 ml) neroli-infused jojoba

1½ oz (42 g) beeswax

7 drops opopanax

2 drops palo santo

3 drops neroli

VETIVER'S
"GROUNDED IN LOVE" PERFUME OIL

Vetiver made this perfume to keep itself feeling grounded in all the love in its life. It never forgets the support of its friends!

Use this recipe: for a natural, earthy, soft perfume.

0.35 oz (10 ml) vanilla-infused jojoba

3 drops vetiver

1 drop bergamot mint

1 drop rose

DIRECTIONS

Make the blend in a 0.35 oz (10 ml) glass roller-top bottle. Pour the vanilla-infused jojoba into the bottle and add the essential oils.

FOR KIDS 🖤

Substitute:

0.35 oz (10 ml) vanilla-infused jojoba

1 drop vetiver

1 drop rose

FRANKINCENSE'S
"MY BODY IS A TEMPLE"
BODY OIL

Frankincense knows when people take care of themselves, they begin to feel their own beauty. It made this body oil to help them do that.

Use this recipe: to moisturize your skin and inspire deep appreciation for your own body.

1 oz (30 ml) jojoba

5 drops spikenard

3 drops neroli

8 drops frankincense

DIRECTIONS

Make the blend in a 1 oz (30 ml) glass bottle. Pour the jojoba into the bottle and add the essential oils.

FOR KIDS 💜

Substitute:

1 oz (30 ml) jojoba

1 drop spikenard

1 drop neroli

4 drops frankincense

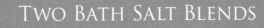
DIRECTIONS FOR BATH SALT BLENDS

Use a 2 oz (60 ml) glass jar for this blend.

Put the salt into the jar. Blend the jojoba and essential oils in a separate bowl before adding to the salt. Stir with a glass stirring rod or the handle of a stainless-steel spoon.

Each recipe makes enough for one bath, though you can make more and store it in a glass jar. The jojoba provides a skin-nourishing carrier to distribute the essential oils.

Pay attention to your skin's responses when using essential oils in a bath. What's comfortable for you may be different from what's comfortable for other people. You may want more jojoba, less essential oil, or different essential oils from the ones in the recipes.

I suggest using about five drops of essential oil total in a bath. When using only floral oils in the recipe, I use even less.

I recommend making these blends fresh every few weeks.

PATCHOULI AND YLANG YLANG'S "SMOOTH HARMONY" BATH SALT

. . . .

Patchouli and Ylang Ylang are the most harmonious pair! They invite you to put on your favorite music, sit back in a warm bath, and let the good vibes take you away.

. . . .

Use this recipe: to wind down in a tub of warm water at the end of the day.

2 oz (56 g) salt

1 teaspoon (5 ml) vanilla-infused jojoba

3 drops patchouli

2 drops ylang ylang

FOR KIDS

Substitute: 2 oz (56 g) salt, 1 teaspoon (5 ml) jojoba, 1 drop patchouli, 1 drop ylang ylang

Meditation and Contemplation

Lavender's "Love the Tub" Bath Salt

Lavender loves relaxing in the tub after a long day . . . or after a peaceful day, or after a busy day, or after a day spent with friends. No matter what kind of day Lavender has, there's no better way to end it than a warm bath.

Use this recipe: for a warm bath that centers you and makes you feel good through and through.

2 oz (56 g) salt

1 teaspoon (5 ml) jojoba

3 drops lavender

2 drops vetiver

FOR KIDS

Substitute:

2 oz (56 g) salt

1 teaspoon (5 ml) jojoba

1 drop lavender

1 drop vetiver

DIRECTIONS FOR INCENSE BLENDS

Put the loose resin in a bowl that holds at least 1 oz (30 ml). Drop the essential oils onto the resin, stirring the loose resin gently with a glass stirring rod or the handle of a stainless-steel spoon. Leave the container open to let the blend dry for about two days, stirring once or twice a day, and then pour it into a 1 oz (30 ml) glass jar with a lid for storage.

To burn the incense, use a heat-safe incense burner and larger-size natural bamboo charcoal. Unlike self-igniting charcoal, natural bamboo charcoal is free of chemicals. It's also free of fragrance and irritants, and reduces environmental pollutants.

Bamboo's extraordinary microstructure makes it highly absorbent when made into charcoal. It's ideal for burning loose incense, wood chips, resins, and herbs. To light the charcoal, hold a tab of it with a small pair of tongs or set the tab up vertically in your incense burner. Hold a flame to the charcoal until it ignites. The bamboo won't spark, but you'll be able to see it is lit when the edge begins smoldering bright red or orange. You can blow on it gently to see the smoldering edge more easily.

Lay the tab of charcoal down in your incense burner and sprinkle a pinch of the loose incense over it. You don't have to get every piece of incense on top of the charcoal. As long as it's touching the charcoal, it will burn.

FRANKINCENSE'S
"IT ALL MAKES SENSE" INCENSE

Nobody understands quite like Frankincense how much it can help to find a calm, reflective place in your mind when you want to figure something out.

Use this recipe: to clear your mind and spend time in reflection.

1 oz (28 g) loose frankincense resin

3 drops frankincense

3 drops palo santo

3 drops opopanax

MYRRH'S
"MAKE THIS ROOM A TEMPLE"
INCENSE

Myrrh loves creating small pockets of beauty everywhere it goes, reminding us of the goodness in everyday life. This incense is one of its favorite blends for making any room feel special.

Use this recipe: to fill the air with a beautiful aroma and create an atmosphere of peace and contemplation.

1 oz (28 g) loose myrrh resin

5 drops spikenard

4 drops frankincense

Natural Cleaning

When people mention they aren't feeling as vibrant or healthy as they would like, one of the first things I ask is whether they're using all-natural cleaning products in their home. I began using natural cleaning products with essential oils in the late 1980s, and I've never looked back!

Simply switching from chemical cleaners to all-natural ones can make such a difference in your health. Surrounding yourself with chemicals in every part of your home can take a lot of your immune system's attention, as it constantly has to work to reduce any reactions that might develop. Replacing those chemicals with natural essential oil cleaners can free up your body's attention to deal with other potential issues. This can increase your vitality and help you feel healthier.

Some people clean with essential oils to calm allergic reactions and asthma. Helping get rid of allergies is one way natural cleaning products have had such a powerful impact on me. It's true that there are potential allergens all around you, but you can use essential oils all around you too! You can bring their supportive presence to kitchen surfaces, bathrooms, tubs and tiles, floors, and more—nearly everything that gets cleaned is an opportunity to use healthy, supportive essential oils.

This chapter includes recipes for natural surface cleaners, tub scrubs, air freshener blends, and more. Essential oils are very effective, and cleaners made with them tend to be gentler if you get them on your skin or inhale them while you're cleaning. In fact, they can support your health. They can help you feel better if you're sick and can clean up your environment so you're less likely to get sick in the first place.

For people who would rather not use chemical cleaners in their homes, essential oil cleaners are wonderful alternatives. For people who are sensitive to chemicals, they can feel like lifesavers! Of course, another benefit is that they make your home smell amazing. You may have to use a little more elbow grease than you would with chemical cleaners, but the results are well worth it.

Before you make any of the following recipes, be sure to check the shelf lives of your ingredients so you know how long your product will last, and any safety concerns for the essential oils.

Tea Tree and Peppermint's "Mold Is Not Invited" Spray

. . . .

Tea Tree and Peppermint love to host big parties (they also love cleaning up after), and they always keep the atmosphere welcoming and fresh. That means mold is not invited.

. . . .

Use this recipe: to help prevent mold from growing.

1 oz (30 ml) tea tree hydrosol

1 oz (30 ml) peppermint hydrosol

4 drops tea tree

4 drops peppermint

DIRECTIONS

Make this blend in a 2 oz (60 ml) glass spray bottle. Pour the hydrosols into the bottle and add the essential oils. Shake before each use.

Spray this blend often anywhere you think mold might want to grow, such as bathrooms and other humid areas. Let it sit for about 15 minutes, and then wipe the area dry.

I recommend making this blend fresh every few weeks.

HEMLOCK'S "A HEALTHY SPACE TO BREATHE" DIFFUSER BLEND

Hemlock loves to create clean environments and healthy spaces to be in. With this diffuser blend it can create healthy spaces to *breathe* in too!

Use this recipe: to cleanse and freshen the air, especially when you want to stay healthy.

6 drops hemlock

4 drops saro

DIRECTIONS

Simply drop the essential oils into the diffuser.

FOR KIDS 💜

Substitute:

3 drops hemlock

2 drops cedarwood

Lavender's "Squeaky Clean Skin-Friendly" Dish Soap

Lavender is a firm believer that keeping a clean, beautiful home goes hand in hand with health and comfort. It doesn't like dish soaps that can irritate skin.

Use this recipe: to clean your dishes by hand at the sink.

6 oz (168 g) castile soap

1 oz (30 ml) lavender hydrosol

12 drops lavender

8 drops rosalina

8 drops tea tree

DIRECTIONS

Make this blend in an 8 oz (240 ml) plastic squeeze bottle. Pour the castile soap and hydrosol into the squeeze bottle, and then add the essential oils. Shake before each use.

I recommend making this blend fresh every few weeks.

LAVENDER AND ORANGE'S "BEAUTIFUL VIEW" GLASS CLEANER

Lavender and Orange want to help you see the world clearly so you'll notice the beauty all around you. That's why they made this glass cleaner for windows (and other glass surfaces).

Use this recipe: to clean glass surfaces.

8 oz (240 ml) water

1 teaspoon (5 ml) vinegar

16 drops lavender

16 drops orange

DIRECTIONS

Make this blend in an 8 oz (240 ml) glass spray bottle. Pour the water and vinegar into the bottle, and then add the essential oils. Shake well, and then spray and wipe glass surfaces clean.

I recommend making this blend fresh every few weeks.

HEMLOCK'S "I LOVE TO CLEAN EVERYTHING" ON-THE-GO ALL-PURPOSE AMAZING KITCHEN AND BATHROOM SPRAY

Hemlock used so many words to name this recipe because it's proud that it can clean so many things! Hemlock even makes a small travel bottle to use when out and about.

Use this recipe: to clean any and every surface in your kitchen and bathroom.

8 oz (240 ml) water

1 teaspoon (5 ml) castile soap

14 drops hemlock

8 drops peppermint

10 drops tea tree

DIRECTIONS

Make this blend in an 8 oz (240 ml) glass spray bottle. Pour the water and castile soap into the bottle, and then add the essential oils. Shake well, spray any surface you'd like to clean, and wipe it dry.

I recommend making this blend fresh every few weeks.

If you'd like to use your favorite hydrosol in this recipe, you can use 2 oz (60 ml) hydrosol and 6 oz (180 ml) water instead of a full 8 oz (240 ml) water. This is a great option because hydrosol adds to the cleaning effects of the blend, and it smells amazing.

LIME'S "CITRUS MINT" BATHROOM SPRITZ

Lime likes every room in its home to be fresh and inviting—even the bathroom. It keeps this blend by the sink and goes through a bottle every week.

Use this recipe: to freshen the air in your bathroom.

2 oz (60 ml) water

5 drops lime

3 drops peppermint

DIRECTIONS

Make this blend in a 2 oz (60 ml) glass spray bottle. Pour the water into the bottle, and then add the essential oils. Shake well and spray into the air in your bathroom.

I recommend making this blend fresh every few weeks.

Lavender's
"Scrub-a-Dub-Dub"
Citrus Tub Scrub

Lavender knows that kitchens and bathrooms can sometimes be tough to clean, but with a combination of this blend and a little elbow grease, it always gets the job done.

Use this recipe: to scrub your kitchen, bathtub, sink, tile, shower, and faucet fixtures.

8 oz (224 g) baking soda

3 tablespoons (45 ml) castile soap

12 drops lavender

9 drops lime

9 drops orange

DIRECTIONS

Make this blend in an 8 oz (240 ml) glass container with a lid. Put the baking soda and castile soap into the container, and mix them with a spoon, creating a paste. Add the essential oils. You can adjust this blend to achieve a consistency you like. More castile soap will give you a smoother paste.

Use a small scoop of the scrub on a sponge to clean your tub and tile.

Lemon's
"Bowl of Fresh Lemons"
Toilet Cleaner

Lemon likes everything to smell very fresh. It loves the aromas of clean laundry, ocean breezes, and just-been-cut grass. It even loves the way the bathroom smells after it uses this recipe.

Use this recipe: to clean and deodorize your toilet bowl.

1 oz (28 g) baking soda

2 drops lemon

DIRECTIONS

You can use the toilet bowl itself as the mixing bowl for this blend. Put the baking soda and lemon essential oil into the toilet bowl, scrub well, and let stand for five minutes. Then flush the toilet and enjoy your fresh bathroom!

LAVENDER'S
"COMFY AND COZY UPHOLSTERY CARE" SPRAY

(#1 OF LAVENDER'S HOME CARE TRIO)

Lavender would love to scent your favorite chair or couch so you can cuddle up in comfort. It promises to take good care of you and offer all the soothing relaxation you could want.

Use this recipe: to freshen your carpets and upholstery.

4 oz (120 ml) lavender hydrosol

DIRECTIONS

Spray the hydrosol onto your upholstery and carpet to help clean it and make it smell beautiful.

You may want to test a small area first to be sure your upholstery likes this spray as much as you do. This spray may not be right for leather or certain fabrics.

Be sure to check with the supplier about the shelf life of your hydrosol.

Lavender's
"Comfy and Clean"
Carpet Care Powder

. . . .

Lavender loves the way clean carpets feel on its bare feet. It uses this carpet powder to keep its own carpets fresh, clean, and inviting.

. . . .

Use this recipe: to give your carpets and rugs a deep deodorizing treatment.

1 oz (28 g) baking soda

1 drop lavender (optional)

DIRECTIONS

You can use 1 oz (28 g) of baking soda alone, and sprinkle it over your carpet or rugs. Let it sit for 15 minutes, and then vacuum.

If you want to add 1 drop of lavender essential oil, mix it into the baking soda in a small bowl before sprinkling it over the carpet. Make sure no pets or small children will come around to roll on the carpet before you vacuum the baking soda blend up.

LAVENDER'S "CLEAN AND CAREFREE" KITCHEN FLOOR CARE

(#3 OF LAVENDER'S HOME CARE TRIO)

. . . .

After Lavender created carpet and upholstery care, it was on a roll! It made an aromatic kitchen floor cleaner that's safe for kids and pets.

. . . .

Use this recipe: to clean your kitchen floor.

8 oz (240 ml) hot water

1 teaspoon (5 ml) vinegar

1 oz (30 ml) lavender hydrosol

DIRECTIONS

If you're using a traditional mop, boil 8 oz (240 ml) water and pour it in a bucket big enough to dip the head of your mop. Pour the vinegar and lavender hydrosol into the water, and mop your floors.

Rather than a traditional mop, you can use a mop with a reusable terry cloth cover, which you can wash and use again. I use a steam mop with a reusable terry cloth cover that provides really hot water for cleaning. It's used like a regular mop, and it works well.

I recommend making this blend fresh every time you mop.

Cedarwood's "Warm and Woodsy" Hardwood Polish

Cedarwood made this recipe to support its friends from the woods. It loves to bring out their best and help them shine!

Use this recipe: to give a lustrous shine to hardwood shelves, tables, and other furniture.

½ oz (14 g) beeswax

2 oz (60 ml) jojoba

10 drops cedarwood

DIRECTIONS

Use a 4 oz (120 ml) glass jar for this blend.

Set up the Stovetop Melting Method (**pages 133–134**). Melt the beeswax in the Pyrex measuring cup. Add the jojoba and remelt. Add the essential oil, stirring gently with a glass stirring rod or the handle of a stainless-steel spoon. Pour the blend into the 4 oz (120 ml) wide-mouth glass jar.

Use a small amount on a soft cloth, rub it into your hardwood surfaces, and then wipe off the excess.

Natural Cleaning

Peppermint and Cedarwood's "No More Sticky Spot" Remover

Peppermint bought a new box to store all of its essential oils, but when it peeled off the label, a spot of sticky goop remained. Cedarwood helped it create this sticky residue remover to clean it up.

Use this recipe: to remove sticky residue from firm surfaces.

1 teaspoon (5 ml) jojoba

1 teaspoon (5 g) salt

1 drop peppermint or cedarwood (optional)

DIRECTIONS

Mix your jojoba and salt in a small bowl. If you'd like to add essential oil, a single drop will do. Peppermint or cedarwood are good choices, because bugs don't seem to like them. However, you can use this as sticky remover without any essential oil at all. Use it for firm surfaces, not upholstery or linen.

There's no need to make a lot of this blend because you won't need to use very much at one time, and you won't need to use it very often. You can make a fresh batch "on the spot" anytime you need it.

LIME'S
"CLEAN IN NO TIME"
SHOWER STALL SPRAY

Lime uses this spray after every shower to keep the shower stall sparkling and fresh. That way soap film, hard water residue, and other grime doesn't have a chance to build up.

Use this recipe: to spray on shower surfaces to prevent soap film and hard water residue from building up.

2 oz (60 ml) water

1 tablespoon (15 ml) vinegar

4 drops lime

2 drops peppermint

2 drops lemon

DIRECTIONS

Make this blend in a 2 oz (60 ml) glass spray bottle. Pour the water and vinegar into the bottle, and then add the essential oils. After you're done showering, shake the shower spray. Then spray the tile, floor, shower door or curtain, and faucet fixtures.

You can leave the blend in the shower for easy access every time you need it. If you'd like to wipe the surfaces down after using the shower spray, keep a sponge with your bottle.

I recommend making this blend fresh every few weeks.

afterword

There is so much to know about essential oils and hydrosols, and the field of aromatherapy is expanding every year. New companies, classes, and conferences are constantly being created, and new research is being done. It's a very exciting time!

Once you grasp the basics of blending your own products and using essential oils safely, the ways aromatherapy can support your own life can keep expanding too. The information and recipes in this book offer you an excellent place to start. You'll also find a few resources for continuing your own learning on the next few pages.

For me, aromatherapy has been a lifelong journey. It has led me to new professional opportunities and wonderful friends, and to beauty I would never have experienced if not for the plants, oils, and amazing people who work with them. I've been on this path for a long time, and it still feels as though there is more to explore.

I feel so honored to share my love of essential oils with you in this book. May it help support your own precious journey!

LEARN MORE ABOUT
AROMATHERAPY AT

Aromahead
Institute

Aromahead Institute offers a rich variety of online classes and webinar tutorials to help expand your understanding of aromatherapy. You can start with Aromahead's popular free class, "Introduction to Essential Oils." (Yes, it's really free!) The class "Aromatherapy for Natural Living" goes deeper into using essential oils in your daily life. The "Aromatherapy Certification Program" offers the training you need to become a certified aromatherapist. Aromahead also offers classes on using aromatherapy for colds and flu, aromatherapy for massage, and more—all on your own schedule and from the comfort of your own home or your favorite coffee shop.

Aromahead's online classes are easy to use and fun! The lessons guide you step by step through reading, watching videos, doing activities, and making blends. The variety of learning styles we incorporate ensure that you're learning on multiple levels and getting hands-on experience.

You'll also be connected with a supportive community of Aromahead Institute students and graduates, and your entire experience will be guided by me and the Aromahead team.

www.aromahead.com

Aromatherapy Resources

Professional Aromatherapy Associations

Alliance of International Aromatherapists (AIA)
www.alliance-aromatherapists.org

International Federation of Professional Aromatherapists (IFPA) www.ifparoma.org

National Association for Holistic Aromatherapy (NAHA)
www.naha.org

Aromatherapy Publications

Alliance of International Aromatherapists Newsletter (USA) • www.alliance-aromatherapists.org

Aromatherapy Today (Australia)
www.aromatherapytoday.com

International Journal of Clinical Aromatherapy (IJCA; France) • www.ijca.net

International Journal of Professional Holistic Aromatherapy (USA)
enhancements.abmp.com/international-journal-of-professional-holistic-aromatherapy

National Association for Holistic Aromatherapy Aromatherapy Journal (USA) • www.naha.org

Essential Oils

Aromatics International, Montana, USA
Aromatics International imports essential oils directly from distillers. Each oil is GC or GC/MS tested. The oils' GC reports are on the website and can be printed. The oils are all organic, wild-crafted, or unsprayed. www.aromatics.com

Essential Elements, Florida, USA
Imports essential oils directly from distillers. Each oil is GC or GC/MS tested. The oils are all organic, wild-crafted, or unsprayed. www.essentialelementssite.com

Florihana Distillery France
Each oil is GC or GC/MS tested. The oils' GC reports are on the website and can be printed. The oils are all organic, wild-crafted, or unsprayed. www.florihana-usa.com

Tours of France

Essential Oil Resource Consultants (EORC)
Rhiannon Lewis, Provence, France
E-mail: essentialorc@club-internet.fr
www.essentialorc.com

Bottles

Aromatics International
Blank inhalers (a rainbow of colors), PET plastic bottles and jars, glass bottles of various sizes and colors. www.aromatics.com

SKS Bottle & Packaging, Inc.
A varied selection of glass and plastic bottles, jars, lip balm tubes, and more. Phone: 518-880-6980
www.sks-bottle.com

Specialty Bottle
A varied selection of glass and plastic bottles and jars. Phone: 206-382-1100 • www.specialtybottle.com

Carriers

Aromatics International
All organic and unrefined: tamanu oil, jojoba wax, shea butter, cocoa butter, beeswax, and many more butters, lotion, and hydrosols • www.aromatics.com

Mountain Rose
Great supplier for carrier oils, dried herbs, and other ingredients for handmade products. www.mountainroseherbs.com

Pink Himalayan Salt

Aromatics International
Course and finely textured pink salt. www.aromatics.com

Real Salt
Course and finely textured pink salt. www.realsalt.com

Trauma Oil
A combination of arnica, St. John's wort, and calendula infused into a carrier oil (usually olive oil).

Aromatics International. • www.aromatics.com

Herb Pharm. • www.herb-pharm.com

Unscented Lotion

Aromatics International. • www.aromatics.com

Elizabeth Van Buren. • www.elizabethvanburen.com

Shea Butter

Agbanga Karite • www.agbangakarite.com

Aromatics International • www.aromatics.com

Coconut Oil

Agbanga Karite • www.agbangakarite.com

Aromatics International • www.aromatics.com

Cocoa Butter

Aromatics International. • www.aromatics.com

Mountain Rose. • www.mountainrose.com

Beeswax

Aromatics International
Organic beeswax pellets. • www.aromatics.com

Charcoal
For burning loose incense

Aromatics International. • www.aromatics.com

Scents of Earth. • www.scents-of-earth.com

Labels for Bottles

Online Labels. • www.onlinelabels.com

Richmark Labels
Blank labels and laminate labels. I use laminate labels that are the same size as the labels I write on. The clear laminate label goes right over the top of the one with my writing on it, so it does not smear.
Phone: 800-456-8884. • www.richmarklabel.com

Glass Stirring Rods and Pouring Beakers

Indigo Instruments. • www.indigo.com

Science Company. • www.sciencecompany.com

Aromahead Institute's Educational Resources

Aromahead's Blog. • www.aromahead.com/blog

Component Database
View molecular structures, chemical families, safety considerations, and therapeutic properties of essential oil components.. • components.aromahead.com

International Directory of Essential Oil Distillers
Buy essential oils directly from distillers around the world. • www.distillerdirectory.com

Monthly Newsletter: Essential News
www.aromahead.com/newsletters

Aromahead Institute's Social Media

Facebook
www.facebook.com/Aromatherapyeducation

Google +
http://bit.ly/GoogleAromahead

Instagram
https://www.instagram.com/aromahead

LinkedIn
www.linkedin.com/in/aromatherapy

Pinterest
www.pinterest.com/aromahead

Twitter
http://twitter.com/aromahead

YouTube
www.youtube.com/user/TrustYourSource

Bibliography

Battaglia, Salvatore. *The Complete Guide to Aromatherapy*, Second edition, 2004, Perfect Potion.

Keville, Kathi and Mindy Green. *Aromatherapy: A Complete Guide to the Healing Art*, Second edtion, 2008, Crossing Press.

Mojay, Gabriel. *Aromatherapy for Healing the Spirit: Restoring Emotional and Mental Balance with Essential Oils*, 2000, Healing Arts Press.

Rhind, Jennifer Peace. *Listening to Scent: An Olfactory Journey with Aromatic Plants and Their Extracts*, 2014, Singing Dragon.

Rhind, Jennifer Peace. *Aromatherapeutic Blending: Essential Oils in Synergy*, 2015, Singing Dragon.

Tisserand, Robert, and Rodney Young. *Essential Oil Safety: A Guide for Health Care Professionals*, Second edition, 2013, Churchill Livingstone.

Aromatherapy Resources

INDEX

Note: Page numbers in *italics* indicate recipes. Page numbers in **bold** indicate profile/summary information (characteristics, uses, safety tips, etc.) of essential oils, carrier oils, and butters.

THE HEART OF AROMATHERAPY

ACKNOWLEDGMENTS

To Leslie: Thank you for continually inspiring me to write and create with an open heart. Collaborating with you brought *The Heart of Aromatherapy* to life. I am grateful for your exceptional editing, our daily laughter, and your presence in my life.

To everyone at Hay House who supported the publishing of this book: thank you for your brilliant guidance. It is a great honor to write for such an enlightened publishing company.

My gratitude to the Aromahead team: Mina Napolitano, Nicole Lauber, Denise Johnston, Shelia Murray, Ann Lohr, Michelle Gilbert, Beth Hornak, Keith Morgan, Dereck Curry, and Rebecca Silence. You are the heart and soul of Aromahead Institute. Thank you for so generously offering your wisdom and support. Who knew work could be this much fun?!

To all Aromahead Institute students and graduates: it is such a pleasure to be on this aromatherapy journey with you. It's incredible to witness the healing you offer to the world, one blend at a time.

To Rhiannon Lewis, Gabriel Mojay, Jennifer Peace Rhind, Robert Tisserand, Ann Harman, Kailash Dixit, Gary Henderson, Melanie McMurrain, Shane Johnston, and Nick Unsworth, and the whole Aromatics International family: I feel very fortunate to have such inspiring teachers and friends. Thank you for sharing your knowledge with such grace and for all the laughter along the way!

The farmers and distillers I've written of here are only a few of the amazing people I've been privileged to know and work with over the years. It's their dedication and love for what they do that makes what we do, as aromatherapists, possible. I feel such gratitude in my heart for them every time I use essential oils. I extend a heartfelt thank-you to all the farmers and distillers doing this work!

My sweet friends, as I travel through each day and explore this world, you live within me, always a comfort: Christina Polnyj Pollman, Curt Pollman, Linda Ruth, Edie Pett, Annie Powell, Peris Gumz, William Horden, Leonor Horden, Liz Fulcher, Karen Williams, Larry Williams, Amy Hausman, Bernadette Fiocca, Rachel Hogencamp, Sandra Hartman, Sally Ryan, Valerie Romanoff, Sue Dozoretz, Brian Dozoretz, Kc Rossi, Kelly Smith, Amy Whitney, Scott Montgomery, Minta Meyer, Terese Miller, Joy Musacchio, Cynthia Brownley, Theresa Crosier, Lee Whitridge, and Pete Whitridge.

To my parents; my sister, Karen; and Judy Butje, thank you for always being here for me. I love you.

ABOUT THE AUTHOR

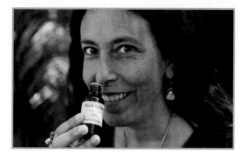

Andrea Butje is an internationally recognized aromatherapist and author. Her aromatherapy school, Aromahead Institute, reaches students from around the world thanks to her innovative online educational programs and her inspired approach to creating community. In 2013, Andrea was honored with a Lifetime Achievement Award from the Alliance of International Aromatherapists for the remarkable work she has accomplished in the aromatherapy profession. You can visit her online at www.aromahead.com.

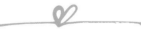

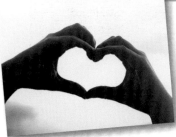
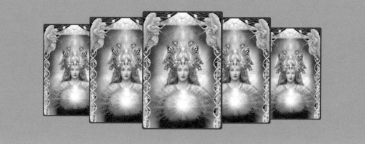